The Pharmacy Tech

Basic Pharmacology and Calculations

Robert Reilly, Pharm. D.
Assistant Director of Pharmacy
Clinical Services
Thomason General Hospital
El Paso, Texas

John Arross, R. Ph.
Staff Pharmacist
Saint Mary's Hospital and Medical Center
Grand Junction, Colorado

Kris Boyea-Sandberg, R. Ph.
Pharmacist
Thomason General Hospital
El Paso, Texas

DELMAR
THOMSON LEARNING

Africa • Australia • Canada • Denmark • Japan • Mexico • New Zealand • Philippines
Puerto Rico • Singapore • Spain • United Kingdom • United States

NOTICE TO THE READER

Publisher does not warrant or guarantee any of the products described herein or perform any independent analysis in connection with any of the product information contained herein. Publisher does not assume, and expressly disclaims, any obligation to obtain and include information other than that provided to it by the manufacturer.

The reader is expressly warned to consider and adopt all safety precautions that might be indicated by the activities herein and to avoid all potential hazards. By following the instructions contained herein, the reader willingly assumes all risks in connection with such instructions.

The Publisher makes no representation or warranties of any kind, including but not limited to, the warranties of fitness for particular purpose or merchantability, nor are any such representations implied with respect to the material set forth herein, and the publisher takes no responsibility with respect to such material. The publisher shall not be liable for any special, consequential, or exemplary damages resulting, in whole or part, from the readers' use of, or reliance upon, this material.

COPYRIGHT © 1994 Delmar, a division of Thomson Learning, Inc. The Thomson Learning™ is a trademark used herein under license.

Printed in Canada
2 3 4 5 6 7 8 9 10 XXX 05 04 03 02 01 00

For more information, contact Delmar, 3 Columbia Circle, PO Box 15015, Albany, NY 12212-0515; or find us on the World Wide Web at http://www.delmar.com

International Division List

Asia
Thomson Learning
60 Albert Street, #15-01
Albert Complex
Singapore 189969
Tel: 65 336 6411
Fax: 65 336 7411

Japan:
Thomson Learning
Palaceside Building 5F
1-1-1 Hitotsubashi, Chiyoda-ku
Tokyo 100 0003 Japan
Tel: 813 5218 6544
Fax: 813 5218 6551

Australia/New Zealand:
Nelson/Thomson Learning
102 Dodds Street
South Melbourne, Victoria 3205
Australia
Tel: 61 39 685 4111
Fax: 61 39 685 4199

UK/Europe/Middle East
Thomson Learning
Berkshire House
168-173 High Holborn
London
WC1V 7AA United Kingdom
Tel: 44 171 497 1422
Fax: 44 171 497 1426

Latin America:
Thomson Learning
Seneca, 53
Colonia Polanco
11560 Mexico D.F. Mexico
Tel: 525-281-2906
Fax: 525-281-2656

Canada:
Nelson/Thomson Learning
1120 Birchmount Road
Scarborough, Ontario
Canada M1K 5G4
Tel: 416-752-9100
Fax: 416-752-8102

ALL RIGHTS RESERVED. No part of this work covered by the copyright hereon may be reproduced or used in any form or by any means—graphic, electronic, or mechanical, including photocopying, recording, taping, Web distribution or information storage and retrieval systems—without the written permission of the publisher.

For permission to use material from this text or product contact us by
Tel (800) 730-2214; Fax (800) 730-2215; www.thomsonrights.com

Library of Congress Cataloging-in-Publication Data
Reilly, Robert / Arross, John/Boyea-Sandberg, Kris
The Pharmacy Tech: Basic Pharmacology and Calculations / Robert Reilly, John Arross, Kris Boyea-Sandberg

1. Allied Health Handbooks, Manuals
2. Medical Handbooks, Manuals

ISBN: 1-56930-005-4

Table of Contents

UNIT I

Basic Pharmacology and Pharmacokinetics

Acknowledgments v

Chapter 1: BASIC PHARMACOKINETICS

Aspects of Pharmacokinetics 2
Absorption 2
Distribution 3
Metabolism 3
Excretion 3

Chapter 2: DOSAGE FORMS

Types of Dosage Forms 5
Routes of Administration 6
Fluid Compatibilities and Incompatibilities 6
Storage of Dosage Forms 7

Chapter 3: BASIC PHARMACOLOGY OF SELECTED DRUG CLASSIFICATIONS

Antihistamines 9
Antimicrobial Drugs 10
Special Anti-infectives 11
Antineoplastic Drugs 12
Anticoagulants 13
Cardiovascular Drugs 14
Antihypertensive Drugs 16
Angiotensins-Converting Enzyme Inhibitors 17
Central Nervous System Drugs 20
Topical Drugs 29
Gastrointestinal Drugs 34
Hormones 38
Muscle Relaxants 44
Vitamins 47

UNIT II

Preparation and Handling of Sterile Products

Chapter 4: PHARMACY-PREPARED STERILE PRODUCTS
Scope of Practice 50
Routes of Administration 50
Methods of Administration 51

Chapter 5: ASEPTIC TECHNIQUE AND STERILE PRODUCT PREPARATION
Theory of Aseptic Technique 53
Laminar Airflow Hoods 54

Chapter 6: PERSONNEL
Education, Training and Evaluation 59
Attire 60
Handwashing 60
Supplies 60

Chapter 7: PROPER HANDLING OF STERILE PRODUCTS
Manipulation of Contents of a ViaL 64
Manipulation of Contents of an Ampule 65
Labeling Requirements 66
Inspecting Final Sterile Product 67
Antineoplastic Medications—Special Considerations 67

UNIT III

Calculations for the Pharmacy Tech

Chapter 8: TIPS FOR PROBLEM SOLVING
The Technician and Pharmacy Math 70
Tips for Successful Problem-solving 71

Chapter 9: THE LANGUAGE OF PHARMACY
Learning the Language 73
Latin Abbreviations and Their Meanings 75

Chapter 10: FRACTIONS
Defining Fractions 78
Enlarging And Reducing Fractions 79
Adding and Subtracting Fractions 81
Multiplying Fractions 82
Dividing Fractions 82
Calculators and Fractions 83

Chapter 11: THE METRIC SYSTEM
Units of Metric Measurement 85
Conversions of Metric Measurement 87

Chapter 12: APOTHECARIES' AND AVOIRDUPOIS SYSTEMS OF MEASUREMENT
Understanding the Systems 89
Conversion of Units of Differing Systems 91

Chapter 13: RATIO AND PROPORTION
Methods of Calculation 94
Ratio and Proportion 96

Chapter 14: ROUNDING
Rules of Rounding 102

Chapter 15: DOSING
Defining Dosing 103
Body Surface Area Dosing 105
Dosing of Tablets and Capsules 108
Dosing of Liquids 108
Dispensing the Various Dosage Forms 111
Constant Infusions 113
Calculating Flow Rates Using Drop Factors 115
Calculating Infusion Rates Based on Hang Time 116

Chapter 16: MISCELLANEOUS CALCULATIONS
Insulin Measurement 120
Temperature Conversion 121
Automatic Compounders 122

Chapter 17: DILUTIONS
Understanding Dilutions 125

Chapter 18: ELECTROLYTE CALCULATIONS
Defining Electrolytes 129
The Milliequivalent 130
Conversions 132
Calculating mEq for Compounds 133
Saline Preparations 134
Preparation of Various Saline Solutions 135

Chapter 19: PERCENTAGE PREPARATIONS
Percent Strength 138
Practical Applications 139
Alligation Method of Calculation 142
Dextrose in Saline Calculations 144

Chapter 20: PHARMACY ECONOMICS
Why Pharmacy Economics? 147
Calculating Percentage Markups 148
Using Fees to Determine Price 149

Answer Key 153
Index 157

Acknowledgements

The authors and publishers of this text would like to thank Tom Lanum, R.Ph. for his contributions to the creation of the chapter on Pharmacy Economics. His efforts are much appreciated.

Special thanks to Anna Maria, Corrine, and Kevin. Without their understanding and support, this project would not have been possible. Also to be thanked is Angie Gerstein for her initiation of this project.

UNIT I

Basic Pharmacology and Pharmacokinetics

Chapter 1
BASIC PHARMACOKINETICS

In this chapter:
- *Absorption*
- *Distribution*
- *Metabolism*
- *Excretion*

ASPECTS OF PHARMACOKINETICS

Pharmacology is the study of the action and effects of drugs on the human body. The drugs described here are used in the prevention and treatment of diseases.

Points to Remember:
- Pharmacokinetics is the study of how the body affects drugs.
- There are four aspects of this:
    - Absorption
    - Distribution
    - Metabolism or biotransformation
    - Excretion

ABSORPTION

Drugs must be absorbed into the body to reach the area where they are required. This can be accomplished several ways. Drugs taken by mouth and swallowed are then absorbed and enter the bloodstream via the digestive system. Drugs may be injected directly into the bloodstream via intravenous (into the vein) or intra-arterial (into the artery) injections using a needle. Intramuscular injections are administered deep into a muscle mass where the drug slowly diffuses into the bloodstream. Intradermal injections are given into the top layer of skin, and subcutaneous injections are administered into the fat layer between the skin and muscle and then diffuse into the bloodstream.

The skin is a very important barrier to infection. Drugs that are injected into the body must be sterile and nonpyrogenic because the skin barrier has been compromised through this form of administration. Sterile refers to the absence of living organisms. However, sterility does not guarantee the fitness of an injectable product. For a product to be appropriate for injectable use, it must also be **nonpyrogenic**. Pyrogens are the bits and pieces of once-living organisms that can trigger the immune system and cause symptoms similar to those of infection: fever, dangerously low blood pressure and changes in metabolism. If a product is nonpyrogenic, then it must be sterile.

Medications may also be inserted into the rectum or vagina or placed into the eyes, nose or ears. These drugs act specifically on the areas where they are placed or diffuse into the bloodstream to reach other areas of the body. Sublingual use of drugs occurs when a drug is placed under the tongue where it dissolves and is absorbed into the bloodstream. Additionally, drugs may be applied to the skin and either act directly on the area of application or form a depot and from there diffuse into the bloodstream.

Each drug has specific characteristics that allow absorption from different routes of administration. Some drugs cannot be given by mouth because they are destroyed by stomach acid. Others cannot be injected because they will not dissolve and transform into a solution suitable for injections into veins and arteries, or they damage the veins or other tissues. For a drug to have a therapeutic effect, it must be absorbed into the body to reach the target area or organ.

DISTRIBUTION

Distribution is the second aspect of pharmacokinetics. Distribution is the process through which the drug travels to the area where it is needed after being absorbed by the body. Some drugs travel throughout the body and penetrate most of the organ systems. Others are more selective and stay in the body water or in the body fat. Certain drugs are able to penetrate the brain in varying degrees. Obviously, for a drug to be of any use in treating or preventing a disease, it must be distributed to the target area. If a drug penetrates fat better than it does any other tissue, that drug is said to be **lipophilic**. Lipophilic drugs also penetrate the brain and other parts of the nervous system better than their lipophobic counterparts.

METABOLISM

Metabolism, or biotransformation, is the third aspect of pharmacokinetics. Although some drugs metabolize differently, metabolism usually takes place in the liver. Metabolism is the process through which the body rids itself of toxins or foreign substances, such as medications. Some drugs are changed chemically eventually inactivated, and then excreted from the body. An interesting variation of this is those drugs that are inactive when absorbed into the body and require metabolism to change them into their active forms. Certain active drugs are also metabolized into other active forms with different chemical properties. Not all drugs undergo metabolism. These drugs are excreted from the body unchanged.

EXCRETION

Excretion is the final aspect of pharmacokinetics. Excretion is the process through which drugs are passed out of the body. Most drugs are excreted by the kidneys and pass out in the urine; others are excreted in bile and through feces, still others leave the body via the lungs during respiration. The kidney is the most important organ for the elimination of drugs. Unchanged drugs or metabolites of drugs are most often excreted by the kidneys.

Proper elimination of drugs is critical. If, for some reason, the liver or the kidneys are not functioning properly, drugs may accumulate in the body and reach toxic concentrations or cause serious side effects. When the liver or kidneys are damaged, the doses of medication generally should be smaller. As a person gets older, kidney and liver function may deteriorate, so smaller doses may be required.

The time it takes to completely rid the body of a drug varies considerably. Half-life is the term used to describe this. The time it takes for the body to rid itself of half of the amount of the drug present in the body is defined as half-life. Four to five half-lives are required to completely rid the body of a drug after the last dose has been given. Some drugs have a very long half-life, and the drug may still be in the body a week or more after the last dose has been given.

Half-life can be used to determine how often to give a dose of a drug. Generally, drugs with a shorter half-life have to be administered more frequently while those with a longer half-life can be administered less frequently.

Chapter 2
DOSAGE FORMS

In this chapter:
- *Types of Dosage Forms*
- *Routes of Administration*
- *Fluid Compatibilities and Incompatibilities*
- *Storage of Dosage Forms*

TYPES OF DOSAGE FORMS

There are many different ways to administer medications. Each route of administration requires a specific dosage form. Drugs taken by mouth and swallowed may be tablets, capsules, chewable tablets, elixirs, solutions or suspensions. Certain tablets may be administered sublingually (allowed to dissolve under the tongue) and are absorbed through the tissue. Drugs may also be inhaled through the mouth or nose.

Certain oral drugs are formulated to be released slowly into the stomach or small intestine. These specific medications are commonly referred to as slow-release or sustained action drugs. They should never be divided or crushed. A dangerously high dose of the drug could be absorbed by the patient over a very short period of time and cause toxicity.

Many medications have an unpleasant, bitter taste which the manufacturer attempts to disguise with a sugar coating. Drugs with this hard outer coating of sugar must not be cut or crushed because to do so would release the bitter flavor.

Dosage forms requiring injection into the body are called parenteral dosage forms. These drugs are most often solutions and suspensions. They are delivered directly into a vein (intravenous) or a muscle (intramuscular). Others are injected into different skin layers (subcutaneous and intradermal), and still others may be injected into the fluid surrounding the brain and spinal cord (intrathecal and epidural).

Solutions and suspensions may also be administered by droppers into the eyes, ears or nose. These drug solutions and suspensions may be placed in spray bottles to be administered into the nose or back of the throat.

Drugs can be added to creams, ointments and lotions and applied to the skin. Ointments may be placed in the eyes. Creams may also be inserted into the rectum or vagina with the use of special applicators. Drugs may be placed in a waxy base and formed into rectal or vaginal suppositories that are inserted into the rectum or vagina.

ROUTES OF ADMINISTRATION

The anatomical site at which the drug enters the body is known as the **route**. The various routes and anatomical sites through which drugs enter the body are outlined in the chart below:

Route	Abbreviation	Anatomical Site
Oral	P.O.	mouth (swallowed)
Sublingual	S.L.	under the tongue
Intramuscular	I.M.	into the muscle
Intradermal	I.D.	into the skin
Subcutaneous	S.C. or S.Q.	under the skin
Intravenous	I.V.	into the vein
Transdermal	T.D	applied to the skin where it is absorbed
Topical	TOP	applied to the skin, little or no absorption
Rectal	P.R.	into the rectum
Epidural	—	into the spinal fluid

FLUID COMPATIBILITIES AND INCOMPATIBILITIES

In dealing with medications in solution, it is very helpful to remember that drugs are chemicals, and that many chemicals react with others if suitable conditions exist.

Incompatibilities can take several forms: The drugs may combine together to form a **precipitate**. Precipitates can be dangerous because they can lodge in the small blood vessels of the lung, thereby preventing absorption of enough oxygen to sustain life. These precipitates may also act as a base around which the blood is able to clot. These clots may travel to the brain or the lungs with disastrous results.

Another type of incompatibility is inactivation of one or both drug products. This inactivation is less dangerous from an immediate perspective, but giving an inactivated drug is the same as not giving any therapy, which may be just as bad for the patient.

A drug combination may not be compatible if it sits in a syringe for several hours or days. However, the drugs may be compatible if they are only to be in contact with each other for a brief period of time. The references available explain under what conditions the compatibility or incompatibility exists. When a drug combination is not listed in the references, that combination has not been studied and should not be recommended for use.

Many questions of compatibility/incompatibility arise not between two drugs but between a drug and the solution with which it is being mixed. A striking example of this is when amphotericin B (an antifungal agent) is mixed with a normal saline (NS) solution. Within a few minutes, a drug complex that looks like snow will form. This complex (called a **colloid**) will occur every time amphotericin B is mixed with NS and should never be attempted. On the other hand, amphotericin mixes well with D_5W and sterile water. An antibiotic combination of trimethoprim and sulfamethoxazole may be mixed with D_5W but must be used within a few hours because the drug loses potency rapidly. A dilute solution of this drug combination is more stable than a more concentrated one. A solution of etoposide in D_5W will form crystals if the solution is too concentrated, and much of the drug will be lost.

Given these examples, the student may ask, "Why do we even attempt dissolving these drugs in these solutions?" The answer is that these drugs can cause serious side effects (severe itching, fever, etc.) if they are given too rapidly. It is impractical to have a nurse stand by the patient for 1-3 hours and slowly push the drug with a syringe.

Given the tremendous number of injectable drugs available, it has become impractical, if not impossible, to memorize all of the compatibilities and incompatibilities that exist. This problem is compounded by the fact that many new injectable drugs are added each year.

As with other aspects of drug therapy, there are reference books available to help with the formidable task of determining if different drug solutions will be compatible. The two most commonly used references are: *The Handbook of Injectable Drugs* (or Trissell's Guide), and *King's Guide to Parenteral Admixtures*. Both references collect data from a multitude of sources on both compatibilities and incompatibilities. It is advantageous to have both references on hand as there are times when compatibility data is listed in one reference, but not the other. Because King's and Trissel's guides are updated frequently, it is very important to receive and keep these updates so as to have the most complete information available.

There are other sources of compatibility information, but few are complete. *Facts and Comparisons*, a complete drug information source, has some compatibility information listed. It should be considered a third backup to search through if Trissel's and King's guides do not have the data being sought. *Facts and Comparisons* is limited in that it only lists large volume solutions (D_5, NS, $D_5\frac{1}{2}NS$, etc.) in which a drug is compatible.

In addition, most pharmacies have developed charts containing common drugs and the solutions with which they are compatible as well as how long they are compatible with those solutions. If the charts do not contain the information sought, King's or Trissel's guides should be consulted.

STORAGE OF DOSAGE FORMS

Proper storage of medications is critical to stability and potency. Many medications require refrigeration; exposure to heat deactivates such drugs. Additionally, refrigeration extends the stability of certain medications. For instance, an antibiotic solution is stable for 24 hours at room temperature but is stable for one week if refrigerated. Light will degrade other drugs, and, as a result, dark bags or storage containers are required. Drug storage areas must maintain proper temperature and humidity to ensure stability of all medications.

Medications must be stored and packaged according to label specifications in order to guarantee the stability and potency of the medication through the manufacturer's labeled expiration date. Failure to adhere to these specifications may result not only in reduced potency, or loss thereof, but may also cause a change in physical appearance of the medication. Physical changes include discoloration, powdered, wet, or crystallized appearance, an unusual smell, or a change in consistency.

The stability of a medication can be influenced by environmental conditions of storage such as temperature, light, air and humidity. Required storage conditions must be included in the labeling of all medications and observed throughout the distribution of the medication to help insure medication potency and stability. The manufacturer's expiration date applies only if these storage requirements are met until the medication is handled through the dispenser or seller to the consumer. The importance of proper storage conditions should be reinforced to the consumer, or patient, at the time of patient counseling. However, it must be recognized that proper control beyond the dispenser or seller is difficult to maintain.

Storage Definitions

The following are storage definitions as defined in the USPXII-NF XVII for recommended conditions commonly specified on medication labels.

Temperature

Freezer: A place in which the temperature is maintained thermostatically between -20°C and -10°C (-4°F and -14°F).

Cold: Any temperature not exceeding 8°C (46°F). A refrigerator is a cold place in which the temperature is maintained thermostatically between 2°C and 8°C (36°-46°F).

Cool: Any temperature between 8°C and 15°C (49°-59°F). Any medication that requires cool storage alternatively may be stored in a refrigerator, unless otherwise specified by required labeling.

Room temperature: The temperature prevailing in a work area.

Controlled room temperature: A temperature maintained thermostatically that encompasses the usual and customary working environment of 20°C to 25°C (68°-77°F) and allows for brief deviations between 15°C and 30°C (59°-86°F) that are experienced in pharmacies, hospitals and warehouses. A medication labeled for storage at "controlled room temperature" may, alternatively, be stored in a cool place, unless otherwise specified by required labeling.

Warm: Any temperature between 30°C and 40°C (86°-104°F)

Excessive heat: Any temperature above 40°C (104°F)

Protection from freezing: Where, in addition to the risk of breakage of the container, freezing subjects a medication to a loss of strength or potency, or to destructive alteration of its characteristics, the container label must bear an appropriate instruction to protect the label from freezing.

Container

Immediate container: A container that holds the medication and is in direct contact with the medication. The container must not interact physically or chemically with the medication so as to alter the strength, quality, or purity of the medication.

Tamper-resistant container: Any container or packaging or a sterile product that is sealed in a manner such that the contents cannot be used without obvious destruction of the seal.

Light-resistant container: Any container that protects the contents from the effects of light by virtue of the properties of the material from which it is made, including any coating applied to it. Labeling indicating to "protect from light" refers to the use of a light-resistant container. When a medication is to be packaged in a light-resistant container and the container is made light-resistant by use of an opaque covering, a single-use or unit dose container may not be removed from the opaque covering until prior to being dispensed.

Well-closed container: Any container that protects the contents from extraneous solids and from loss of contents under ordinary conditions of handling, shipment, storage and distribution.

Tight container: Any container that protects the medication from contamination from extraneous solids, liquids or vapors from loss of contents and evaporation, liquification or crystallization under ordinary conditions of handling, shipment, storage and distribution.

Hermetic container: Any container that is impervious to air or other gas under ordinary conditions of handling, shipment, storage and distribution.

Chapter 3
BASIC PHARMACOLOGY OF SELECTED DRUG CLASSIFICATIONS

In this chapter:
- *Selected Drug Groups*
- *Common Actions and Side Effects*
- *Brand and Generic Names for Selected Drugs*

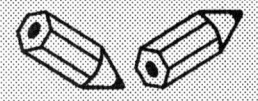

The purpose of this chapter is to familiarize the pharmacy technician with common drugs and to provide basic information about these medications. The drugs listed here have been grouped according to their uses. Listed under each type of drug are the generic and, in most cases, the common brand names. The common side effects are highlighted in each group.

ANTIHISTAMINES

Antihistamines are used to treat the symptoms of allegery such as sneezing, watery eyes and itching. Histamine is one of the chemicals released in the body that causes these symptoms, and the antihistamine drugs block the histamine effect on the body. Common antihistamine drugs are listed by generic or chemical name.

GENERIC	TRADE
astemizole	Hismanal®
chlorpheniramine maleate	Chlor-Trimeton®
dimenhydrinate	Dramamine®
diphenhydramine HCl	Benadryl®
hydroxyzine HCl	Atarax®, Vistaril®
meclizine HCl	Antivert®
promethazine HCl	Phenergan®
terfenadine	Seldane®

Uses

These drugs may be used in combination with decongestants (agents that relieve nasal congestion or stuffy nose). They are also useful in treating some types of dizziness and motion sickness. In addition, promethazine and hydroxyzine are commonly used to prevent or treat nausea associated with the administration of narcotics such as meperidine (Demerol®).

Because the itching and watery eyes of allergies are often accompanied by nasal congestion, pharmaceutical manufacturers have marketed products which combine an antihistamine with a decongestant. Some common products and their components are listed below.

Antihistamine/Decongestant Combinations

BRAND NAME	ANTIHISTAMINE	DECONGESTANT
Actifed®	triprolidine	pseudoephedrine
Dimetapp®	brompheniramine	phenylpropanolamine
Drixoral®	dexbrompheniramine	pseudoephedrine
Ornade®	chlorpheniramine	phenylpropanolamine

Dosage Forms

Tablets, capsules, elixir, syrup, and sustained-release tablets and capsules

---

✜ SIDE EFFECTS:

Drowsiness; stomach upset

ANTIMICROBIAL DRUGS

Anti-infective drugs are used to treat different kinds of infections. These drugs are also called antibiotics or antimicrobial agents. Infections are caused by living, one-celled microorganisms such as bacteria, fungi and viruses. The anti-infective drugs stop or slow the growth of these organisms by breaking down the organism's cell wall or by not allowing the organisms to multiply. Common anti-infective drugs used to treat bacterial infections are:

GENERIC	TRADE
• amoxicillin trihydrate	• Amoxil®
• ampicillin	• Omnipen-N®
• aztreonam	• Azactam®
• cefazolin sodium	• Kefzol®
• cefotaxime sodium	• Claforan®
• cefoxitin sodium	• Mefoxin®
• ceftriaxone sodium	• Rocephin®
• cefuroxime sodium	• Zinacef®
• cephalexin	• Keflex®
• co-trimoxazole	• Bactrim,® Septra®
• doxycycline	• Vibramycin®
• erythromycin	• Eryc®, E-mycin®
• gentamicin sulfate	• Garamycin®

GENERIC	TRADE
imipenem	Primaxin®
metronidazole	Flagyl®
nafcillin sodium	Unipen®
neomycin/polymyxin	Neosporin®
penicillin	Veetids,® Pen-vee K®
piperacillin sodium	Pipracil®
tetracycline HCl	Sumycin®
ticarcillin disodium	Ticar®
tobramycin sulfate	Nebcin®
vancomycin HCl	Vancocin®

Uses

Anti-infective drugs may be effective against specific organisms, and use of more than one drug is common in treating certain infections.

SPECIAL ANTI-INFECTIVES

Antifungal agents may be administered intravenously, orally, applied topically or inserted into the rectum or vagina to treat infections caused by fungi (yeasts) such as *Candida albicans*. Fungi are present everywhere and are slow-growing; therefore, it is very difficult to contract a fungal infection because the immune system will normally eradicate the fungus before it has a chance to grow. However, once established, the fungus may be difficult to kill, and treatment may last many weeks. Common anti-infective agents used to treat fungal infections are:

GENERIC	TRADE
amphotericin B	Fungizone®
clotrimazole	Lotrimin®
fluconazole	Diflucan®
griseofulvin	Fulvicin®
ketoconazole	Nizoral®
miconazole	Monistat®
nystatin	Mycostatin®
tolnaftate	Tinactin®

Other Anti-infectives

Viral infections are extremely difficult to treat and there are fewer antiviral agents than other anti-infective agents. Common antiviral drugs are:

GENERIC	TRADE
acyclovir	Zovirax®
didanosine (DDL)	Videx®
ribavirin	Virazole®
vidarabine	Vira A®
zalcitabine, (DDC)	Hivid®
zidovudine, (AZT)	Retrovir®

Uses

The above drugs work against only a few types of viruses, none of which causes the common cold. Rimantadine and amantadine will prevent certain strains of flu if taken very soon after symptoms start. Acyclovir has activity against the herpes virus if given during the outbreak; it has no activity against a dormant virus. Acyclovir also works against *Varicella zoster* and cytomegalovirus.

Ribavirin kills the respiratory syncytial virus, a life-threatening lung infection that strikes primarily children and the elderly. Zalcitabine, didanosine and zidovudine affect the human immunodeficiency virus (HIV). These drugs do not halt the progression of the infection, but they do slow it down for a period of time. Vidarabine is active against only the herpes virus. Because it may promote liver tumors if used systematically, this drug is confined primarily to topical use.

Dosage Forms

Antibiotics may be administered orally, intravenously, intramuscularly, topically on the skin, in the eyes and ears, in the vagina, injected intrathecally and sometimes instilled into the urinary bladder.

✣ SIDE EFFECTS:

Stomach upset, rashes, diarrhea; may damage the kidneys and liver

ANTINEOPLASTIC DRUGS

Antineoplastic drugs are prescribed to treat different types of cancers. These drugs are also called chemotherapeutic agents or chemotherapy. Because the term "cancer" actually covers hundreds of different diseases, the use of antineoplastic drugs varies a great deal depending on the type of cancer being treated. In addition, other drugs may be mixed with antineoplastics to treat the common side effects.

The more common antineoplastic agents are:

GENERIC	TRADE
• bleomycin sulfate	• Blenoxane®
• busulfan	• Myleran®
• carboplatin	• Paraplatin®
• chlorambucil	• Leukeran®
• cisplatin	• Platinol®
• cyclophosphamide	• Cytoxan®
• cytarabine	• ARA-C®
• dacarbazine	• DTIC®
• daunorubicin	• Cerubidine®
• doxorubicin	• Adriamycin®
• fludarabine phosphate	• Fludara®
• 5-fluorouracil	• 5-FU
• idarubicin	• Idamycin®
• ifosfamide	• Ifex®
• methotrexate	• Folex®
• mitomycin	• Mutamycin®

GENERIC	TRADE
• mitoxantrone	• Novantrone®
• paclitaxel	• Taxol®
• tamoxifen	• Nolvadex®
• vinblastine sulfate	• Velban®
• vincristine sulfate	• Oncovin®

Dosage Forms

Antineoplastic agents are most often given intravenously, though selected agents are given orally.

✢ SIDE EFFECTS:

Severe bone marrow suppression in which the body cannot produce white blood cells to fight infections. Hair loss and nausea or vomiting are also common. Open, painful sores may develop in the mouth and anus.

One of the difficulties in treating cancer is that tumors are composed of abnormal cells which rapidly multiply. Drugs cannot differentiate between a cancer cell and a normal cell. As a result, antineoplastic drugs kill both normal and abnormal cells, and are, therefore, very toxic. Chemotherapeutic agents attack rapidly multiplying normal cells such as hair cells, skin cells, bone marrow cells, and the cells lining the mouth, stomach, intestines and anus, thus, resulting in the most common side effects.

The side effects associated with these drugs are managed by a variety of means. The sores that develop in the mouth are normally treated with mouthwash mixtures composed of antihistamines, local anesthetics and thickening agents that cause the other ingredients to adhere to the sores long enough for them to work. Sores outside the body are treated primarily with frequent cleansing and dressing changes but may also include local anesthetics. The bone marrow suppression created by these compounds is treated by limiting exposure to bacteria and by giving injections of filgrastim (Neupogen), a compound that stimulates bone marrow production of white blood cells.

Nausea and vomiting are frequent side effects of these medications and are generally treated with one or more of the drugs listed below:

GENERIC	TRADE
• droperidol	• Inapsine®
• granisetron	• Kytril®
• metoclopramide HCl	• Reglan®
• ondansetron HCl	• Zofran®
• prochlorperazine	• Compazine®
• promethazine	• Phenergan®
• trimethobenzamide HCl	• Tigan®

ANTICOAGULANTS

Anticoagulants are drugs used to decrease coagulation or clotting of the blood. These drugs are also called "blood thinners". Blood clotting is a normal reaction to stop bleeding when injury occurs. However, clots in the blood vessels may break loose and lodge in the vessels of the heart, lungs or brain and there cause serious damage or even death. Heart attacks are often caused by blood clots blocking the vessels of the heart, and some strokes are caused by

14 *Basic Pharmacology*

clots blocking vessels in the brain. Whenever blood vessels are blocked, the tissue surrounding that area dies.

Common Anticoagulants

Heparin and warfarin (Coumadin®) are the two most commonly used anticoagulants.

A new anticoagulant, enoxaparin (Lovenox), is used primarily after joint replacement procedures to prevent clot formation around the new joint. Enoxaparin acts similarly to heparin.

Warfarin works by preventing the creation of coagulation factors that rely on Vitamin K. Because it takes several days to deplete all the Vitamin K dependent factors from the body, this drug does not take full effect immediately. Therefore, Warfarin is often used with Heparin.

The therapeutic effect of warfarin is measured by **prothrombin time** (PT). The PT is measured by the number of seconds it takes a patient's blood to clot under specific circumstances. This value is then compared to a control value. For a therapeutic effect to be observed, the PT must be somewhere between 1.2-2 times the control value.

A more accurate method of measuring warfarin therapy is the **International Normalized Ratio** (INR). This test is much more consistent than the Prothrombin time, and its use is becoming widespread. Normal INR values range from 2-4.5 times control.

Heparin achieves its anticoagulant effect by blocking the activation of clotting factors rather than preventing their formation. Therefore, the drug's onset of action is very nearly immediate. Heparin is available only as an injectable dosage form. The therapeutic effect of Heparin is measured by **Activated Partial Thromboplastin Time** (aPTT). Like the PT, the aPTT is measured in seconds. Generally the aPTT should be between 1.5-2.5 times the control value. The appropriate dose of Heparin is largely determined by trial and error. The drug seems to work best and have fewest side effects when given by continuous infusion. It is, however, often delivered by the subcutaneous route. Heparin is never to be given intramuscularly, because it interacts with the rich supply of blood to the muscle and causes localized bleeding known as a **hematoma**.

Dosage Forms

Heparin must be given intravenously or subcutaneously. Warfarin is available only as an oral tablet in this country.

✥ SIDE EFFECTS:

Prolonged bleeding; **Possible cause:** Overmedication or use of other drugs that interact negatively

CARDIOVASCULAR DRUGS

Cardiovascular drugs are used to treat problems of the cardiovascular system. The cardiovascular system consists of the heart and all of the blood vessels. The heart contains four chambers—two atria and two ventricles. These chambers contract in a specific sequence to push blood into the lungs and throughout the body. The blood vessels include arteries, veins and capillaries. Arteries carry blood with oxygen to the tissues throughout the body, and veins carry blood with carbon dioxide back to the heart and lungs. Capillaries are tiny blood vessels between the veins and arteries where oxygen and carbon dioxide transfer takes place.

Digoxin

(Lanoxin®, Lanoxicaps®)

Digoxin is a drug used to treat congestive heart failure or atrial fibrillation. In congestive heart failure the heart cannot pump strongly enough for sufficient oxygen-rich blood to reach the tissues. The heartbeat is weak and rapid. Atrial fibrillation occurs when the atria beat very rapidly and out of sequence. Digoxin causes the heart to beat more powerfully and more slowly to allow blood to reach the tissues.

Digoxin is eliminated by the kidneys; therefore, the function of the kidneys should be evaluated before starting therapy. Doses range from 10-60 micrograms per kilogram of body weight depending on the dosage form, the age of the person, kidney function and disease state. Infants and children often receive the drug twice daily because their kidneys can eliminate it very quickly. Adults receive digoxin once daily.

Serum levels are often drawn to determine if too much or too little of the drug is being administered. Such levels may be inaccurate if the patient has more or less muscle than the average individual, as the digoxin concentrates in muscle.

Dosage Forms

Digoxin is available in injectable, tablets, capsules and elixir dosage forms. As each dosage form is absorbed at a different rate and to a different extent, they cannot be easily interchanged.

✢ SIDE EFFECTS:

Heartbeat can be slowed too much. **Lesser side effects:** Diarrhea; vision changes

Because the side effects from digoxin may be dangerous, this drug must be used with extreme caution. Patients should be meticulously monitored because the range between the therapeutic dose and the toxic dose is very narrow.

Antiarrhythmics

Antiarrhythmics are drugs that treat arrhythmias or irregular heartbeats. Some arrhythmias can cause the heart to stop beating while others have very mild effects. Common antiarrhythmics are:

GENERIC	TRADE
• amiodarone HCl	• Cordarone®
• disopyramide	• Norpace®
• encainide	• Encaid®
• flecainide	• Tambocor®
• lidocaine HCl	• Xylocaine®
• mexiletine HCl	• Mexitil®
• procainamide HCl	• Pronestyl, Procan SR®
• quinidine	• Quinidex®

Dosage Forms

The antiarrythmics are available as capsules, IV infusions, tablets, and injectables. Lidocaine has many forms which are used for other purposes.

✜ SIDE EFFECTS:

Stomach upset; diarrhea; more arrhythmias.

Antiarrhythmics must be given cautiously as these drugs may cause other arrhythmias as dangerous as those they are used to treat.

Error prevention alert: Quinidine is a very commonly used antiarrhythmic. It is also is very similar in spelling and pronunciation to quinine, a drug used to treat leg cramps.

ANTIHYPERTENSIVE DRUGS

Hypertension, or high blood pressure, is a common and potentially devastating chronic disease which results in blood being pushed through the vessels at increased pressure. Often, medication must be taken continuously as the diagnosis is made. Several different classes of medications are used to treat hypertension.

Diuretics

Diuretics or "water pills" are drugs that cause the body to lose water, thereby reducing the volume of the blood the heart must pump. This decreases the pressure. Common diuretics are:

GENERIC	TRADE
bumetanide	Bumex®
furosemide	Lasix®
hydrochlorothiazide	Esidrix®
methyclothiazide	Enduron®
spironolactone	Aldactone®
triamterene	Dyrenium®

Of the commonly-used diuretics, only bumetanide and furosemide are available as injectable dosage forms. The other diuretics are available in oral forms.

✜ SIDE EFFECTS:

Stomach upset, frequent urination, potassium depletion, dizziness. **Note:** Spironolactone and triamterene may cause the accumulation of too much potassium.

The most potent diuretics tend to waste the most sodium and potassium; therefore, they are often combined with weak diuretics that conserve potassium. Triamterene is the potassium-sparing diuretic which is most commonly used. Spironolactone is another commonly used potassium-sparing diuretic.

Beta-Blockers

Beta-blockers are also used to treat hypertension. They act by slowing the beating of the heart which causes less blood to be pumped. Common beta-blockers are:

GENERIC	TRADE
atenolol	Tenormin®
esmolol HCl	Brevibloc®
metoprolol tartrate	Lopressor®
nadolol	Corgard®

GENERIC	TRADE
• propranolol	• Inderal®
• timolol maleate	• Blocadren®

Dosage Forms

All of the beta-blockers are available as tablets. Atenolol, metoprolol, and propranolol are also available as injections.

The beta-blockers are metabolized by the liver when they are first absorbed. Therefore, when these drugs are given intravenously a much smaller dose is used.

✣ SIDE EFFECTS:

Slowed heartbeat, profound low blood pressure, dizziness, depression, drowsiness and some stomach upset. **Patients with lung disease:** Some of these drugs can also cause shortness of breath and wheezing. Because these drugs may aggravate asthma, they should not be given to the asthma patient unless no other class of drug can be used.

ANGIOTENSIN-CONVERTING ENZYME INHIBITORS

Another class of drugs for treatment of hypertension is the angiotensin-converting enzyme inhibitors (ACE inhibitors). Angiotensin II is a substance produced in the body that causes the blood vessels to constrict or get smaller. This vasoconstriction causes the blood pressure to increase. The ACE inhibitors block the conversion of angiotensin I to angiotensin II so the blood vessels remain relaxed. ACE inhibitors are:

GENERIC	TRADE
• benazepril	• Lotensin®
• captopril	• Capoten®
• enalapril maleate	• Vasotec®
• fosinopril	• Monopril®
• lisinopril	• Zestril®
• ramipril	• Altace®

Uses

The A.C.E. inhibitors represents a major advance in hypertension therapy. These drugs have fewer side effects than traditional hypertension medications, and they seem to be very effective in preventing the unwanted consequences of hypertension.

However, they are not effective for all patients. If the actions of angiotensin are not the primary contributing factors for the hypertension, the chances of the ACE inhibitors working are diminished.

Dosage Forms

The ACE inhibitors are available primarily in the oral form. The only injectable ACE inhibitor available is enalapril (Vasotec IV), which is the active metabolite of the oral ACE inhibitor enalapril (Vasotec). Ramipril (Altace) is supplied as a capsule, while the rest appear as tablets.

SIDE EFFECTS:

Profound low blood pressure; taste abnormalities; dry cough; blood cell abnormalities; some kidney problems

Calcium-Channel Blockers

The calcium-channel blocking agents are used to treat hypertension as well. All muscles (including the smooth muscles of the blood vessels) need calcium to contract. The calcium-channel blocking agents block the entrance of calcium into the muscle so the muscle does not contract. This, in turn, relaxes the blood vessels and, subsequently, reduces the blood pressure. Some calcium-channel blocking agents are listed below:

GENERIC	TRADE
amlodipine	Norvasc®
bepridil HCl	Vascor®
diltiazem	Cardizem®
felodipine	Plendil®
isradipine	DynaCirc®
nicardipine HCl	Cardene®
nifedipine	Procardia®, Adalat®
verapamil HCl	Calan®, Isoptin®

Uses

These medications are more likely to be effective in the treatment of hypertension occurring in African-Americans and the elderly.

Dosage Forms

Diltiazem (Cardizem®) is the only calcium-channel blocker available in IV form. Felodipine, verapamil, amlodipine, and bepridil are available as tablets. Isradipine and Cardene are available only as capsules. Nifedipine is available as a capsule or sustained release tablet. Verapamil is also available as a sustained-release tablet or capsule. Diltiazem is available in a variety of dosage forms: injectable, tablet, sustained release tablet (for dosing every 12 hours) and controlled delivery (CD) for dosing once per day.

SIDE EFFECTS:

Dizziness, flushing, headache, profound low blood pressure, swelling of the legs and feet, constipation and stomach upset

Vasodilating Agents

Vasodilating agents are another group which specifically dilate, or relax, the blood vessel. Dilated blood vessels allow more blood to flow through, and this causes reduction in blood pressure. Some of these agents are listed below:

GENERIC	TRADE
hydralazine HCl	Apresoline®
isosorbide dinitrate	Isordil®
isosorbide mononitrate	Monoket®, Ismo®

GENERIC	TRADE
• minoxidil	• Loniten®
• nitroglycerin	• Nitrostat®
• papaverine HCl	• Pavabid®

Uses

The vasodilating agents hydralazine and minoxidil are very rarely given as the sole therapy for high blood pressure as their effects are generally short-lived when administered alone. Because the human body has a marvelous capacity to adapt to change, the vasodilators are easily circumvented. As the vasodilator works, blood pressure drops in a dilated blood vessel because there is not enough blood volume to fill the blood vessel. The body can compensate for this by retaining enough fluid to fill the vessel sufficiently to raise the blood pressure again.

Nitroglycerin, isosorbide dinitrate, and isosorbide mononitrate are used primarily for control of angina (chest pain caused by clogged arteries) but can also be used for blood pressure control under certain circumstances such as myocardial infarction (heart attack). These drugs, collectively referred to as nitrates, decrease blood pressure and chest pain by dilating both veins and arteries. Tolerance to their effects can develop quickly when these drugs are administered around the clock. For this reason, a **nitrate-free period** of about 10-12 hours between the last and first doses of the day is recommended.

Dosage Forms

Nitroglycerin is available as an injection, sublingual tablet, translingual (spray), transmucosal (buccal) tablet, sustained release tablet, sustained release capsule, transdermal patch and transdermal ointment. Isosorbide mononitrate and isosorbide dinitrate are available as tablets and sustained release tablets. Isosorbide dinitrate is also available as a sustained-release capsule. Hydralazine is manufactured as a tablet and as an injection. Minoxidil is available as a tablet for the treatment of hypertension. A topical solution of this drug (Rogaine) is marketed as a treatment for male pattern baldness.

✥ SIDE EFFECTS:

Headache and facial flushing

Centrally-Acting Agents

The final group of drugs used to treat hypertension is the centrally-acting agents. These drugs act directly in the brain to change the signals sent to the heart and blood vessels. Some of these agents are listed below:

GENERIC	TRADE
• clonidine HCl	• Catapres®
• doxazosin maleate	• Cardura®
• guanabenz acetate	• Wytensin®
• methyldopa	• Aldomet®
• prazosin HCl	• Minipress®

Uses

Uses far from their original indications have been discovered for some of these drugs. Clonidine, for example, is sometimes used to curb withdrawal symptoms in recovering drug and alcohol abusers. Terazosin is often used to treat benign prostatic hypertrophy (BPH), the medical term for an enlarged prostate. Terazosin and doxasozin make it easier for patients suffering from this condition to urinate because they relax the muscles of the bladder neck and prostate.

Although, the first few doses of prazosin, terazosin or doxazosin can lead to a dramatic decrease in blood pressure, often to the point where the patient may faint, this effect wears off after the first few doses.

Dosage Forms

As it is difficult to achieve the proper dose with the above agents, they are generally reserved for patients who fail other therapies or who would benefit from these drugs' secondary effects on the prostate. These agents are varied in their side effect profiles: the newer agents appear to be better tolerated. Most of these are available in oral forms; methyldopa is also available as an injectable.

✣ SIDE EFFECTS:
Drowsiness; depression; profound low blood pressure

CENTRAL NERVOUS SYSTEM DRUGS

The central nervous system comprises the brain and spinal cord. The brain controls all of the actions of the body. Basically, drugs which act on the central nervous system either stimulate or depress its functions.

Pain is a useful signal to the body that something is wrong, but the pain itself may interfere with healing and normal function. There are two main classes of medications used to treat pain. These groups are the nonsteroidal anti-inflammatory agents and the opiates.

Nonsteroidal Anti-Inflammatory Agents

The nonsteroidal anti-inflammatory drugs (NSAIDs) act by blocking prostaglandins, the substances in the body that cause inflammation and pain. The anti-inflammatory effects of the NSAIDs are exerted outside the central nervous system. However, two effects of the NSAIDS are exerted inside the central nervous system—antipyretic (fever-reducing) and analgesic (pain-reducing). The result is that pain is reduced in two areas.

In patients with fever; these agents act on the hypothalamus (the part of the brain that controls body temperature) to cause vasodilation, which lowers body temperature by radiating heat into the surrounding air. Some of the nonsteroidal anti-inflammatory agents are listed below:

GENERIC	TRADE
• aspirin	• Bayer®
• diclofenac	• Voltarin®, Cataflam®
• diflunisal	• Dolobid®
• etodolac	• Lodine®
• codeine	
• ibuprofen	• Motrin®, Advil®, Rufen®, Pedia-Profen®, Children's Advil®
• indomethacin	• Indocin®
• ketoprofen	• Orudis®
• ketorolac	• Toradol®

GENERIC	TRADE
• oxaprozin	• Daypro®
• piroxicam	• Feldene®
• naproxen	• Anaprox®, Anaprox DS®, Naprosyn®, Aleve®
• salsalate	• Salsitab®, Salflex®, Disalcid®
• magnesium salicylate/choline salicylate	• Trilisate®
• sulindac	• Clinoril®
• tolmetin sodium	• Tolectin®

Uses

Aspirin was the first of these compounds to be discovered and still enjoys widespread use despite competition from the newer anti-inflammatories. Aspirin has been demonstrated to have many uses other than just as a pain blocker. For example, taking aspirin can decrease the risk of having a heart attack. This beneficial effect is the result of the actions of aspirin on platelets. Platelets are the initiators of blood coagulations. Heart attacks are often caused when blood clots inside blood vessels break off and travel to the heart. Once inside the heart, these clots block the smaller arteries feeding the heart, thus shutting off the blood supply. Without oxygen, the section of the heart dies, which leads to a heart attack. Because aspirin makes it more difficult for platelets to stick together, it decreases the patient's chances of having a heart attack.

Ibuprofen (Motrin® and others) also has enjoyed widespread usage because of its over-the-counter (OTC) status. It does not have as strong an effect on platelets as aspirin, but is very effective at relieving pain, inflammation and fever. It is also not as likely to cause stomach ulcers as aspirin and many of the other NSAIDS.

No one NSAID will work for everyone. Persons experiencing chronic pain may be treated with several different drugs before the best one is found.

Dosage Forms

Aspirin is available in a tremendous variety of dosage forms; in fact, the only forms in which it is not available are liquid, injection and topical. Ibuprofen is available in tablet form. Indomethacin (Indocin®) is available as an injectable, but not for the treatment of pain. Injectable indomethacin is used to close the ductus arteriosus; a hole that exists between the ventricles of the heart in the fetus, but should not exist after the baby is born. If the ductus arteriosus does not close soon after birth, the baby's heart cannot pump blood efficiently enough to sustain life. Ketorolac (Toradol®) is one of the few NSAIDs available as an injection for the treatment of pain.

✣ SIDE EFFECTS:

Stomach upset; drowsiness; kidney problems. **Long-term users:** Use with caution as these drugs can cause stomach ulcers.

The Opiates

The opiates are also used for pain. These are powerful drugs that bind to specific places in the brain so that pain is no longer felt. Some of the opiates are listed on the following page.

GENERIC	TRADE
morphine	Astramorph®, Duramorph®, MSIR®, MS Contin®
hydromorphone HCl	Dilaudid®
meperidine	Demerol®
codeine	
propoxyphene HCl	Darvon®, Darvocet® (contains acetaminophen)
fentanyl citrate	Sublimaze®
alfentanyl HCl	Alfenta®
nalbuphine HCl	Nubain®
butorphanol tartrate	Stadol®
pentazocine HCl	Talwin®
oxycodone HCl	Percocet®, Percodan®

Uses

Although the opiates serve a useful function in relieving pain, all of these drugs are habit-forming if abused. When used to treat severe pain; the risk of addiction is small. Generally, patients on long-term opiate therapy will develop tolerance to the drugs effects. When tolerance develops, increasing amounts of drug are needed to treat the patients pain. It is not uncommon for a terminally ill cancer patient to receive doses of morphine large enough to kill a person who has never been given morphine before. Many of the opiates are combined with aspirin or acetaminophen to enhance their pain-blocking effects.

Dosage Forms

The opiates are available in a wide variety of dosage forms including tablets, capsules, oral solutions, rectal suppositories, injectables and IV and IM infusions.

✣ SIDE EFFECTS:

Drowsiness, stomach upset, constipation; an overdose of any of the above drugs can lead to slowed breathing, coma and even death.

Acetaminophen

Acetaminophen, more commonly known by the brand name Tylenol®, is also used to treat pain, but it differs chemically from the nonsteroidal anti-inflammatory drugs and the opiates. Acetaminophen and the nonsteroidal anti-inflammatory agents also reduce fever.

Although acetaminophen can block the pain associated with an injury, it cannot decrease any inflammation that may be present. Acetaminophen does not upset the stomach or cause ulcers as do the NSAIDs.

Dosage Forms

Because acetaminophen is used and marketed widely in this country, any table of dosage forms of this drug would become quickly outdated. The drug is available as tablets, capsules, caplets, gel caps, drops, suspension and effervescent tablets. This drug is also found in combination with just about every antihistamine and decongestant available. It is commonly combined with opiates to enhance their effects.

✤ SIDE EFFECTS:
An overdose of acetaminophen can cause liver failure and even death.

Anticonvulsants

Other agents that work in the central nervous system are used to prevent seizures or convulsions, although their methods of action are not entirely understood. Some of the anticonvulsants are listed below:

GENERIC	TRADE
carbamazepine	Tegretol®
clonazepam	Klonopin®
diazepam	Valium®
divalproex	Depakote®
felbamate	Felbatol®
gabapentin	Neurontin®
phenobarbital	Phenobarbital®
primidone	Mysoline®
phenytoin	Dilantin®
valproic acid	Depakene®

Uses

Tegretol is commonly used as an anticonvulsant as well as in certain types of headaches and psychiatric disorders.

Phenobarbital and primidone are related drugs; primidone is metabolized to phenobarbital plus another compound in the body. The parent compound and both metabolites have anticonvulsant activity.

Clonazepam and diazepam are both benzodiazepines. Diazepam is used primarily in acute care settings because of its prompt onset of activity. However, the drug is not recommended for maintenance therapy because of its short duration of effect. Clonazepam is used for maintenance therapy but it stops working in a significant number of patients (about 30%) after only a few months of therapy.

Divalproex and valproic acid are related compounds; divalproex is a compound formed by linking valproic acid and sodium valproate together; once in the body, they separate and exert their anticonvulsant effects. The drug is also used in the treatment of bipolar disorder.

All of the drugs interact strongly with many other medications; it also tends to be difficult to find an initial stable, effective dose that is not toxic.

For many years there were no new additions to the arsenal of epilepsy treatment. However, in late 1993 and early 1994, two new drugs were released which appear promising—felbamate and gabapentin. Although neither of these agents is perfect; they represent an advance in that they have fewer drug interactions and their side effects are generally milder. These agents are primarily used concurrently with other anticonvulsants. They allow smaller doses of other drugs to be given, which lessens the chance that those drugs will cause side effects.

In the treatment of epilepsy, no one drug works for all, and many patients take several drugs at once to keep symptoms at bay. Therefore, more anticonvulsant drugs being brought to market represents the ability to help more patients control their seizures.

Dosage Forms

While phenytoin is available as tablets, capsules, injection and suspension, these dosage forms are not interchangeable. The tablets release all of their drug immediately, as does the injection and suspension. However, the capsules dissolve slowly and release their drug over an extended period of time. While the capsules, tablets and injection all contain the sodium salt of phenytoin, the suspension contains the free acid form. This makes the suspension more potent than the other dosage forms by about 8%.

Most of these drugs, including carbamazepine, clonazepam, diazepam, valproic acid and primidone are available as tablets. Diazepam is also available as extended release capsules and as an injectable product. Phenobarbital is available in tablet, capsule, elixir and injectable forms.

✣ SIDE EFFECTS:

Drowsiness; stomach upset. Phenytoin can also cause overgrowth of the gum tissue.

Antidepressants

Antidepressant agents are used to treat major depression. These drugs work by altering the abnormal chemicals in the brain that are causing the depression. They may take three to four weeks to take effect.

There are two chemicals present in the human brain which are thought to be responsible for depression when they are deficient—these chemicals are norepinephrine and serotonin. It is not fully understood which one of these chemicals (called **neurotransmitters**) is more responsible for depression.

The drugs used in the treatment of depression act by causing a build up of one or both of the neurotransmitters in the **synapse** (the gap between two nerve cells), or by increasing the nerve cells' sensitivity to neurotransmitters.

There are four types of antidepressant drugs: the tricyclic compounds (TCA's), monoamineoxidase inhibitors (MAOI's), serotonin-uptake inhibitors, and drugs with an unknown mechanism of action.

Monoamine Oxidase Inhibitors

GENERIC	TRADE
• isocarboxazid	• Marplan®
• phenelzine	• Nardil®
• tranylcypromine	• Parnate®

Uses

The MAOI's were the first class of compounds developed for depression. These drugs work well for depression, but have some dangerous side effects.

Dosage Forms

All of the above drugs are available in tablet form only.

✣ SIDE EFFECTS

A patient taking an MAOI must carefully monitor his or her diet for tyramine, an amino acid. Tyramine is present in many foods that have been smoked, aged or fermented. If a person taking an MAOI ingests tyramine, his or her blood pressure can become so elevated as to be life-threatening. Because it is so difficult to follow this diet, these drugs are not commonly used.

Tricyclic Antidepressants

The tricyclic antidepressants (TCA's) were the next discovered. They cause a buildup of both serotonin and norepinephrine.

GENERIC	TRADE
amitriptyline	Elavil,® Endep®
amoxapine	Asendin®
clomipramine	Anafranil®
desipramine	Norpramin®, Pertofrane®
doxepin	Adapin®, Sinequan®
imipramine	Tofranil®, Janimine®
maprotiline	Ludiomil®
nortriptyline	Aventyl®, Pamelor®
protriptyline	Vivactil®
trazodone	Desyrel®
trimipramine	Surmontil®

Uses

In addition to their function as antidepressants, these drugs also have antihistamine and anticholinergic effects.

Dosage Forms

Most of the drugs in this category are available in tablet or capsule form. Only amitriptyline and imipramine are available in injectable forms.

✥ SIDE EFFECTS:

Sedation, dizziness, dry mouth, and urinary retention

Serotonin-Uptake Inhibitors

Serotonin-uptake inhibitors are a relatively new class of compounds. These drugs are very selective in blocking the reabsorption of serotonin by nerve cells, causing a build up of the neurotransmitter in the synapse. The serotonin-uptake inhibitors have a great deal fewer side effects than the other antidepressants.

GENERIC	TRADE
fluoxetine	Prozac®
paroxetine	Paxil®
sertraline	Zoloft®

Bupropion (Wellbutrin®) is chemically unrelated to any other antidepressant. Its mechanism of action is unknown.

26 *Basic Pharmacology*

Dosage Forms

Paroxetine and sertraline are available in tablet form only; fluoxetine is available as capsules and in liquid form.

✜ SIDE EFFECTS:

Drowsiness; constipation; vision changes

Psychotropic Agents

The psychotropic agents are a classification of drugs that act on the central nervous system. These drugs are used to help people with schizophrenia and other mental disorders. These agents include:

GENERIC	TRADE
chlorpromazine	Thorazine®
clozapine	Clozaril®
fluphenazine	Prolixin®
haloperidol	Haldol®
lithium	Lithobid®
loxapine	Loxitane®
mesoridazine	Serentil®
perphenazine	Trilafon®
prochlorperazine	Compazine®
risperidone	Risperdal®
thioridazine	Mellaril®
thiothixene	Navane®
trifluoperazine	Stelazine®

Uses

Lithium (Lithobid®, Lithane®) is the chemically simplest agent available. It is effective for bipolar disorder (manic-depression), but the patient's heart must be monitored before the drug can be started, and patients must be careful to prevent dehydration because this compound can cause heart problems. Blood levels of this drug must be closely monitored during initiation of therapy and periodically after a constant dose has been determined.

Clozapine (Clozaril®) is very effective in the treatment of schizophrenia—a complex disorder having multiple classifications that is beyond the scope of this text. Most schizophrenics are withdrawn and some hallucinate; clozapine decreases the severity of these symptoms. The primary drawback to this medication is the need for weekly blood tests.

Clozapine can cause a potentially fatal blood abnormality called agranulocytosis—a condition in which a component of the immune system is severely depressed, making it difficult for the body to fight off infection. The incidence of this side effect is low (about 1.3%), but continuous monitoring is necessary because it can be fatal.

Haloperidol (Haldol®) is used extensively in the treatment of psychosis. Psychosis has a complex nebulous definition, but these people are generally agitated, depressed, out of touch with reality, and may harm themselves or others in their disturbed emotional state. (Schizophrenia is a type of psychosis.) As with the other antipsychotics, haloperidol decreases the symptoms of psychosis, but does not cure the disorder. The antipsychotics as a group can have some troubling effects on movement. These side effects, called extrapyramidal symptoms or EPS, consist of tremors, changes in posture, alterations in gait and protrusion of the tongue.

There are a multitude of psychotropic agents available and no one drug is effective for everyone. Often a patient will try several different drugs before finding one which will control symptoms adequately and have minimal side effects.

Dosage Forms

Most of these agents are available in oral and injectable forms; clozapine, lithium and thioridazine are available in oral forms only.

✤ SIDE EFFECTS:

Drowsiness; stomach upset; low blood pressure

Benzodiazepines/Barbiturates

The benzodiazepines and barbiturates are agents used to treat anxiety and insomnia and to control seizures. They bind to certain areas of the brain that control anxiousness and wakefulness.

Some commonly used benzodiazepines are listed below:

Benzodiazepines

GENERIC	TRADE
alprazolam	Xanax®
chlordiazepoxide	Librium®
diazepam	Valium®
flurazepam	Dalmane®
lorazepam	Ativan®
midazolam	Versed®
oxazepam	Serax®
temazepam	Restoril®
triazolam	Halcion®

Uses

The benzodiazepines are very safe agents, especially when they are compared to other agents used for seizures, anxiety and insomnia. In overdose situations these agents are rarely fatal unless they are combined with other drugs.

When used in the treatment of insomnia, these agents are effective for short-term use only. If used on a daily basis for more than a few weeks, their effectiveness diminishes. The benzodiazepines should only be used on an as-needed basis because the sleep they produce does not exactly mimic natural sleep in that the period of R.E.M. sleep (a stage of sleep characterized by rapid eye movements) is shortened. Continuous R.E.M. sleep deprivation makes people irritable and less able to concentrate.

This effect of R.E.M. sleep is not significant when the agents are used only occasionally because incomplete sleep is much better than no sleep at all.

Barbiturates

GENERIC	TRADE
• amobarbital	• Amytal®
• pentobarbital	• Nembutal®
• phenobarbital	• Phenobarbital®
• secobarbital	• Seconal®

Uses

The barbiturates are not as safe as the benzodiazepines; therefore, they must be used with greater care. Phenobarbital is used most commonly in the treatment of seizures disorders, generally in combination with other agents.

Pentobarbital is sometimes used in the treatment of insomnia because of its rapid onset of action and rapid clearance from the body. Like the benzodiazepines, all the barbiturates alter the length of time spent in R.E.M. sleep and are effective for only a few weeks. Pentobarbital is also used commonly for induction of general anesthesia because of its rapid onset and clearance.

Dosage Forms

Most of the benzodiazepines and barbiturates are available in tablet and capsule form; chlordiazepoxide, diazepam, lorazepam, midazolam, phenobarbital, pentobarbital, amobarbital, and secobarbital are available as injectable and oral forms.

✣ SIDE EFFECTS:

Drowsiness; memory loss; overdose can cause slowed breathing, coma and even death.
Note: The barbiturates are used infrequently in the general population for anxiety and insomnia.

Stimulants

Stimulants also affect the central nervous system. Some of the stimulants are listed below:

GENERIC	TRADE
• dextroamphetamine	• Dexedrine®
• methylphenidate	• Ritalin®

Uses

These drugs were used in the past as "diet pills" and "uppers", but addiction and abuse were problems. Presently, stimulants are used to treat hyperactive children. One would think that stimulants such as these would make children more active, but children experience the opposite effect.

Dosage Forms

Dextroamphetamine is available in tablets, capsules, elixir and sustained release capsules; methylphenidate is available in tablets and sustained release tablets.

✣ SIDE EFFECTS:

Rapid heartbeat, agitation, high blood pressure, dependency

TOPICAL DRUGS

Several groups of medications are administered to the eyes, ears, nose and throat. Generally these drugs are used for their local effects on the area to which they are administered. Anti-infective agents are used for infections in the eyes or ears. The anti-inflammatory agents are used to treat inflammation of the eyes, ears or nose. Local anesthetics are used to numb areas that are painful. Red eyes and runny noses are treated with vasoconstrictors. Miotics are used to make the pupil of the eye smaller, while mydriatics are used to make the pupil of the eye larger. The different groups of medications with selected agents are listed:

Eye Products

Agents for glaucoma

GENERIC	TRADE
epinephrine	Glaucon®
dipivefrin	Propine®
apraclonidine	Iopidine®
carteolol	Ocupress®
levobunolol	Betagan®
betaxolol	Betoptic®
timolol	Timoptic®
metipranolol	Optipranolol®
acetylcholine	Miochol®
carbachol	Isopto-Carbachol®
pilocarpine	Isopto Carpine®
physostigmine	Isopto Eserine Solution

Anti-infective agents

GENERIC	TRADE
bacitracin	AK-Tracin®
erythromycin	AK-mycin®
gentamicin	Garamycin®
neomycin/polymyxin	Ocutricin®
chloramphenicol	Chloromycetin®
tobramycin	Tobrex®
tetracycline	Achromycin®
ciprofloxacin	Citexan®

Steroidal anti-inflammatory agents

GENERIC	TRADE
dexamethasone	Maxidex®
prednisolone	Pred-Mild®, Inflamase Forte®

Non-steroidal anti-inflammatory agents

GENERIC
- flurbiprofen
- diclofenac
- ketorolac

TRADE
- Ocufen®
- Voltaren®
- Toradol®

Local anesthetic

GENERIC
- proparacaine
- tetracaine

TRADE
- Alcaine®
- Pontocaine®

Vasoconstrictors

GENERIC
- epinephrine
- naphazoline
- oxymetazoline
- phenylephrine
- tetrahydrozoline

TRADE
- Adrenalin Chloride
- Naphcon Forte®
- OcuClear®
- Neo-synephrine®
- Visine®

Mydriatics

GENERIC
- pilocarpine atropine
- cyclopentolate
- dipivefrin
- epinephrine
- homatropine
- phenylephrine
- scopolamine
- tropicamide

TRADE
- Atropisol®
- Cyclogyl®
- Propine®
- Mytrate/Epifrin®
- AK-Homatropine®
- Neo-Synephrine®
- Isopto Hyoscine®
- Mydriacyl Ophthalmic®

Miotics

GENERIC
- acetylcholine
- carbachol
- echothiophate
- isoflurophate
- physostigmine
- pilocarpine

TRADE
- Miochol®
- Miostat®
- Phospholine®
- Floropryl®
- Isopto-Eserine®
- Pilocar®

Tear replacement preparations
- Cellufresh®
- Celluvise®
- Hypotears®
- Liquifilm Forte®

(These products contain various combinations of water, thickening agents, preservatives, vitamins and salts to mimic the hydrating, lubricating and antiseptic actions of tears.)

Ear Preparations

GENERIC	TRADE
neomycin/polymyxin B/hydrocortisone	Cortisporin Otic®
benzocaine/antipyrine	Auralgan®
hydrocortisone/acetic acid	VoSol HC Otic®
acetic acid in aluminum acetate	Burow's Otic®
carbamide peroxide	Debrox®
isopropyl alcohol/glycerin	Swim-ear®
chloramphenicol	Chloromycetin Otic®

Mouth and Throat

GENERIC	TRADE
nystatin	Mycostatin®
tannic acid	Zilactin®
clotrimazole	Mycelex®
chlorhexidine gluconate	Peridex®
carbamide peroxide	Debrox®
benzocaine and cetylpyridinium	Cepacol®
dextromethorphan hydrobromide	Sucrets®
phenol/menthol	Cepastat®
menthol	Vicks Throat®
benzocaine/phenol	Anbesol®

Topical Products for Skin Application

GENERIC — TRADE

Acne

GENERIC	TRADE
tretinoin	Retin-A®
benzoyl peroxide	Desquam-X10®
tetracycline	Topicycline®
erythromycin	A/T/S®
clindamycin	Cleocin T®

Burns

GENERIC
- nitrofurazone
- silver sulfadiazine

TRADE
- Furacin®
- Silvadene®

Dandruff

GENERIC
- selenium sulfide
- coal tar

TRADE
- Selsun Blue®
- Tegrin Medicated®

Miscellaneous

GENERIC
- diphenhydramine/calamine

TRADE
- Caladryl®

Antiviral

GENERIC
- acyclovir

TRADE
- Zovirax®

Antibiotic

GENERIC
- mupirocin
- gentamicin
- polymyxin B/bacitracin
- polymyxin B/neomycin/bacitracin

TRADE
- Bactroban®
- Garamycin®
- Polysporin®
- Neosporin Ointment®

Anti-fungal

GENERIC
- miconazole
- ciclopirox olamine
- tolnaftate
- nystatin

TRADE
- Micatin®
- Loprox®
- Tinactin®
- Nilstat®

Anti-Scabies

GENERIC
- lindane
- permethrin

TRADE
- Kwell®
- Nix®

Steroidal anti-inflammatory agents

GENERIC	TRADE
• augmented betamethasone	• Diprolene®
• betamethasone	• Diprosone®
• clobetasol propionate	• Temovate®
• fluocinolone	• Synalar®
• fluocinonide	• Lidex®
• hydrocortisone	• Hytone®
• triamcinolone	• Aristocort A®

Local anesthetics

GENERIC	TRADE
• benzocaine	• Dermoplast®
• dibucaine	• Nupercainal®
• tetracaine	• Pontocaine®
• lidocaine	• Xylocaine®

Emollients

GENERIC	TRADE
• vitamins A and D/zinc oxide/lanolin	• Desitin®

Skin protectant

GENERIC	TRADE
• aluminum sulfate/calcium acetate	• Domeboro®
• trolamine salicylate	• Myoflex®
• keratolytic	
• salicylic acid	• Compound W®
• podophyllum resin	• Podofin®

Uses

Some of these drugs have no effect when they are taken orally because the liver and kidneys do a very effective job of eliminating them. Often, these drugs are applied topically because the medication would not reach the desired area if taken by mouth or injected.

The technique used to apply these topical products largely determines the effectiveness of the product. Eye drops should be applied only after the hands are washed. The tip of the dropper never should touch the eye and the drop should fall onto the inside of the lower eyelid. If multiple drops are to be applied to the eye, a small amount of time (about 5 minutes) should be allowed before applying the second drop. This should be done because there is only room for one drop on the eye at any one time.

Technique is important for ear drops also. Wet a cotton ball with the drug solution, instill the drops into the ear, then insert the cotton ball gently into the ear. This allows the drug to stay in contact with its site of action for an extended period of time.

When a topical product is to be applied to the skin, the area should be cleaned before a thin layer of product is applied. Thicker layers offer no therapeutic advantage over thin layers and are much messier. Many drugs, especially the steroidal anti-inflammatories and liniments should not be covered with any kind of occlusive dressing (a bandage that will not let air in or out). Doing this can cause burns or severe irritation to the area.

The agents for glaucoma prevent increased intraocular pressure (IOP), which is the cause of glaucoma. Although the liquid inside the eye ball (aqueous humor) is constantly being produced, the normal eye has a drainage system that allows excess aqueous humor to drain from the eye. In the patient suffering from glaucoma, this drain is blocked causing the build-up of fluid inside the eye. The increased pressure that results can damage the optic nerve causing vision loss. Glaucoma drugs act to either decrease the amount of aqueous humor that is produced or to increase the rate of exit of aqueous humor from the eye. Some patients with glaucoma are eventually treated with surgery, but many respond well to drugs.

Even though these drugs are not swallowed or injected, they may have systemic effects because of absorption through the conjunctiva (the area of the eye from which tears appear).

Dosage forms

The availability of forms varies widely from drug to drug. Available forms for the topical drugs listed above include solutions, tablets, ointments, creams, powders and sprays.

✤ SIDE EFFECTS:

Local irritation of the eye, ear, nose or throat; temporary vision changes (mydriatics); ointments may cause briefly blurred vision.

Patients should wear eye protection before going out into the sun and drive only when vision returns to normal.

The topical drugs are popular because of their safety relative to the side effects these same drugs cause when taken internally. Many of the drugs used topically are very toxic when swallowed or injected.

GASTROINTESTINAL DRUGS

The gastrointestinal system is composed of the mouth, esophagus, stomach, small and large intestines, rectum and anus. Gastrointestinal disorders include stomach upset, ulcers, diarrhea, constipation, cramping and vomiting. There are several classes of drugs used to treat these disorders.

Antacids

Antacids are used to treat stomach upset or acid indigestion, and sometimes ulcers. They work by neutralizing the stomach acid. Common antacids include:

GENERIC	TRADE
• aluminum carbonate	• Basaljel®
• aluminum hydroxide	• AlternaGEL®, Amphojel®
• aluminum and magnesium combinations	• Maalox®, Mylanta®, Gaviscon®, Gelusil®, Di-Gel®
• aluminum phosphate	• Phosphaljel®
• calcium carbonate	• Tums®
• dihydroxyaluminum sodium carbonate	• Rolaids Antacid®

GENERIC	TRADE
• magaldrate	• Riopan®
• magnesium hydroxide	• Milk of Magnesia®
• potassium and sodium bicarbonate	• Alka-Seltzer®
• sodium bicarbonate or baking soda	

Simethicone, or Mylicon®, is an agent used to help with painful gas. Often it is combined with the above agents.

Dosage Forms

Available forms for the above agents include tablets, capsules, chewable tablets.

✤ SIDE EFFECTS:

Constipation; diarrhea

Unfortunately most of these products have a chalky taste or a bitter salty taste that is not always masked by the flavoring agents.

Products containing magnesium tend to cause diarrhea while aluminum-containing products are generally constipating. Many products mix the two salts in an effort to decrease the effects of each. Generally, one side effect will dominate but will not be as intense as if that salt had been used alone. Magaldrate contains magnesium and aluminum in the same compound. While this does decrease the amount of diarrhea or constipation observed, it is not as effective and may cause rebound hyperacidity. Calcium containing antacids and magaldrate can cause a condition known as rebound hyperacidity. After these drugs neutralize stomach acid, the stomach is stimulated to produce even more acid, which can cause a return of symptoms.

Antidiarrheals

Medications used to treat diarrhea or frequent watery stools work by either slowing the movements of the intestines or by adding bulk to the stool. Common antidiarrheals are:

GENERIC	TRADE
• diphenoxylate HCl with atropine sulfate	• Lomotil®
• kaolin and pectin	• Kao-Spen®
• loperamide HCl	• Imodium®
• opium	

Kaolin and pectin decrease diarrhea by absorbing liquid and normalizing motility by its physical presence.

Paregoric, opium, loperamide, and diphenoxylate with atropine decrease diarrhea by decreasing the rate and strength of intestinal contractions as well as by decreasing the amount of liquid secreted in to the colon.

Dosage Forms

These products are available in oral forms; diphenoxylate with atropine is available in tablet form only.

✤ SIDE EFFECTS:

Constipation; drowsiness

The liquid products in this category may have an unpleasant taste.

Laxatives

Constipation is the infrequent passing of hard dry stools. Laxatives are agents used to soften the stool or to increase the movements of the intestines to promote passing of stool. Common laxatives and stool softeners are:

GENERIC	TRADE
bisacodyl	Dulcolax®
cascara sagrada	
castor oil	
docusate calcium	Sulfalax Calcium®
docusate sodium	Colace®
magnesium citrate	
magnesium hydroxide	Milk of Magnesia®
methylcellulose	Citrucel®
mineral oil	
phenolphthalein	Ex-Lax®
psyllium	Metamucil®
senna	Senolax®

Uses

Methylcellulose and psyllium are referred to as bulk-forming laxatives. Their mechanism of action is to stimulate intestinal contractions by absorbing liquids and swelling. Bulk-forming laxatives can also be used to treat diarrhea because of their ability to absorb liquid.

Docusate sodium, docusate calcium and mineral oil allow the stool easier passage because of a softening or lubricating agent. Magnesium citrate and magnesium hydroxide are referred to as saline laxatives because they attract and retain water in the colon, which makes evacuation easier. Phenolphthalein, castor oil, bisacodyl, senna and cascara sagrada are the stimulant laxatives. These agents work by irritating the intestinal tract, thus increasing the rate and strength of contraction.

The bulk-forming laxatives can take several days to achieve their effects. Plenty of water should be drunk during therapy to prevent intestinal obstruction and to allow the products to work. These products should not be started in large doses because a painful amount of gas can be produced. Instead, therapy should be started with small doses and the dose increased slowly.

Dosage Forms

Most of these drugs are available in oral forms, but some have other dosage forms available as well. Bisacodyl and senna are available as suppositories while mineral oil and docusate sodium are available as enemas. Phenolphthalein and psyllium are available as chewable products.

✣ SIDE EFFECTS:

Diarrhea; severe cramping with some stimulant laxatives; bowel dependence on the laxative for normal function resulting from overuse. **Note:** Profuse diarrhea can lead to dehydration and electrolyte imbalances.

H₂ Antagonists

Several medications are effective in healing ulcers. The H₂-antagonists inhibit the action of a special type of histamine receptor present in the stomach. This reduces gastric acid production. Listed below are several H₂-antagonists:

GENERIC	TRADE
• cimetidine	• Tagamet®
• famotidine	• Pepcid®
• nizatidine	• Axid®
• ranitidine	• Zantac®

Uses

Sucralfate, or Carafate®, binds to the ulcer site and acts as a protectant. Misoprostol, or Cytotec®, is a drug used to treat or prevent ulcers resulting from the use of nonsteroidal anti-inflammatory agents. Omeprazole, or Prilosec®, is a powerful antiulcer drug that works by stopping the production of stomach acid altogether.

Dosage Forms

The above drugs are available in tablets and injectable form. Cimetidine and ranitadine are additionally available as liquids, and famotidine is available as a powder.

✣ SIDE EFFECTS:

Primarily mild for many drugs; liver problems (rarely); confusion in elderly patients; constipation (Sucralfate); diarrhea (Misoprostol)

Antiemetics

The last group of gastrointestinal agents are the antiemetics or drugs used to decrease nausea and vomiting. These agents affect the vomiting center in the brain. Common antiemetics include:

GENERIC	TRADE
• dimenhydrinate	• Dramamine®
• meclizine	• Antivert®
• ondansetron	• Zofran®
• prochlorperazine	• Compazine®
• promethazine	• Phenergan®
• trimethobenzamide	• Tigan®

Metoclopramide, or Reglan®, is another agent used to treat nausea. It may also be used to stimulate gastrointestinal movements to enhance digestion.

Most of these drugs in this category were developed for different applications. For instance, dimenhydrinate, meclizine, and promethazine are antihistamines and prochlorperazine is an antipsychotic.

Dosage Forms

Dimenhydrinate, promethazine and trimethobenzamide are available as tablets, injectables, and suppositories. Ondansetron is available in injectable form, meclizine is available in tablets, and prochlorperazine is available as tablets, extended release capsules, oral solution and as an injectable product.

✥ SIDE EFFECTS:

Drowsiness, movement disorders, dry mouth

HORMONES

The next large group of drugs is the hormones and synthetic substitutes. The adrenal steroids, sex hormones, insulin, and thyroid hormones are included in this class.

Corticosteroids

The adrenal hormones, or corticosteroids, are drugs with powerful anti-inflammatory effects. The body uses these substances to deal with everyday stresses. Some of the corticosteroids are listed below:

GENERIC	TRADE
betamethasone	Celestone®
dexamethasone	Decadron Phosphate®
fludrocortisone acetate	Florinef Acetate®
flunisolide	AeroBid®
hydrocortisone	Solu-Cortef®
methylprednisolone	Solu-Medrol®
prednisolone	Prelone®
prednisone	Deltasone®
triamcinolone	Aristocort®

Uses

In addition to their anti-inflammatory effects, these drugs have other actions which are used therapeutically. **Mineralocorticoid** effects cause the body to retain water, sodium, potassium and other minerals. Because of this property, Florinef® is used to maintain normal blood pressure in the patient suffering from Addison's disease. The patient with Addison's disease has no ability to conserve sodium and water naturally, so the drug must be given continuously for the life of the patient. **Glucocorticoid** effects impact on the body's ability to mobilize glucose (a sugar) from body stores to supply extra fuel during times of peak need. Hydrocortisone has high glucocorticoid effects. Hydrocortisone is combined with fludrocortisone to treat Addison's disease because Addison's patients do not mobilize glucose efficiently.

Betamethasone is used to accelerate the maturation of fetal lung tissue when it is apparent that the mother has gone into labor too soon and the labor cannot be stopped.

Because of its potent anti-inflammatory effects, methylprednisolone is used in the treatment of asthma. Asthma is a disease in which the lung tissues become inflamed and can swell shut. The airways usually remain open either by themselves or with the help of inhaled corticosteroid and bronchodilators such as theophylline (Theo-Dur®) and albuterol (Proventil®). However, the inflammation will sometimes return and cause an acute attack. Often, injectable methylprednisolone will be used to decrease the swelling to the point where the patient can breathe.

Additionally, methylprednisolone is used to treat spinal cord injuries. Although this use is relatively new, this drug has preserved the ability to walk in thousands of spinal cord injury patients. As with any other tissue, when the spinal cord is injured, an inflammatory response is initiated. This reaction brings nutrients, oxygen and immune system components to the site of injury quickly. However, this response also brings swelling; and since the cord is encased in the spine, in the past, the resulting pressure often damaged the cord. Methylprednisolone in extremely high doses is used to stop the inflammatory response before this damage can occur. If the therapy is initiated in time, many patients will regain nearly full mobility.

Dosage Forms

Betamethasone, dexamethasone, prednisolone and triamcinolone are available in tablet and injectable forms. Additionally, dexamethasone is available as an elixir and an oral solution. Fludrocortisone is available in tablet form while prednisone is available as tablets and oral solution. Hydrocortisone is available in many forms including ointments, lotions, sprays and creams; methylprednisolone is available as an ointment. Flunisolide is available as a nasal solution.

✥ SIDE EFFECTS:

Stomach upset. **Long-term use:** *Weight gain* resulting from increased appetite. *Fat* deposited around the face ("moon face"), on the back between the shoulder blades ("buffalo hump") and in other places. *Dependency* as the adrenal glands may stop producing these substances which will result in problems if the drugs are stopped too suddenly. *Inability* of the body *to properly handle sugars* and *cholesterol*.

Sex Hormones

Another group of steroids, the sex hormones, can be divided into androgens (male sex hormones), estrogens (female sex hormones) and progestins. These substances are important for the development and function of the sexual organs and are necessary for normal pregnancy and birth. Some of the common androgens are listed below:

Androgens

GENERIC	TRADE
danazol	Danocrine®
fluoxymesterone	Halotestin®
testosterone	Andro 100®

Uses

The androgens are used to treat delayed puberty and males who don't develop normal testicular function. They have recently been used in studies trying to reestablish vigor in elderly males who have limited mobility. They are also used illegally by many athletes in an effort to increase athletic performance.

Dosage Forms

Danazol is available in capsule form; fluoxymesterone is available in tablets. Testosterone is an injectable product.

SIDE EFFECTS:
Masculinization; increased facial and body hair; deepened voice; acne; aggressive behavior

Estrogens

Some of the common estrogens are listed below:

GENERIC	TRADE
dienestrol	Ortho Dienestrol®
diethylstilbestrol	Stilphostrol®
estradiol	Estrace®, Estraderm®, Depo Estradiol®
estrogenic substances, conjugated	Premarin®
quinestrol	Estrovis®

Uses
The estrogens are primarily used to decrease bone loss in post-menopausal women. Estrogens also decrease the frequency and severity of hot flashes as well as the amount of vaginal dryness experienced by post-menopausal women. Doses higher than those used for menopausal symptoms are used in the treatment of abnormal uterine bleeding, female hypogonadism, and prostatic carcinoma.

Dosage Forms
All of these drugs are available in tablet form. Additionally, diethylstilbestrol is available as vaginal suppositories, dienestrol is available as vaginal cream and estradiol is an injectable.

SIDE EFFECTS:
Feminization; stomach upset; depression; some increased blood clotting

Progestins

Some of the common progestins are listed below:

GENERIC	TRADE
medroxyprogesterone acetate	Provera®
megestrol acetate	Megace®
norethindrone	Norlutin®

Uses
The progestins are used in combination with estrogens in the treatment of menopause. The presence of the progestin decreases the risk of endometrial hyperplasia and possibly cancer. Progestins are used alone in the treatment of amenorrhea, abnormal uterine bleeding and endometriosis.

Dosage Forms
All three of these drugs are available in tablet form; additionally, medroxyprogesterone is available in an injectable form.

✢ SIDE EFFECTS:

Stomach upset; depression; liver failure and cancer (androgens), high blood cholesterol (androgens)

Oral Contraceptives

The oral contraceptives or "birth control pills" are combinations of estrogens and progestins. Some of the oral contraceptives are listed below:

- Brevicon®
- Ortho-Cept®
- Ovral®
- Demulen®
- Ortho-Novum®
- Triphasil®

Uses

Both estrogen and progesterone are produced by the body and function to regulate the menstrual cycle. It may seem contradictory to use compounds that cause maturation, release and implantation of the egg in the prevention of conception. However, these compounds make very effective contraceptives. While the body requires high levels of estrogen and progesterone to prepare the uterus for pregnancy and cause the actual release of the egg, there is also a need for low levels of both hormones to allow the hypothalamus to release follicle-stimulating hormone-releasing factor (FSH-RH). This releasing factor stimulates the initial growth of the follicle in the ovary that contains the egg.

Combination oral contraceptives deliver enough estrogen daily to prevent the release of FSH-RH. They also contain enough of a progesterone-like compound during the latter part of the cycle to create an inhospitable environment for sperm and to disrupt the critical time sequence needed for implantation in the uterus. Basically, the birth control pill fools the body into thinking it is pregnant when it really is not.

Dosage Forms

As the name implies, oral contraceptive are available in oral forms.

✢ SIDE EFFECTS

Circulatory complications, nausea, missed menses, breast tenderness or fullness (in some women), headaches, increased risk of liver tumors (rare), spotting or breakthrough bleeding

Insulin

Insulin is a natural hormone produced by the pancreas that controls the use and storage of sugars. Diabetes is the disease in which either too little insulin is produced or no insulin is produced at all. If no insulin is produced by the pancreas, the body must receive insulin in order to survive. Insulin is obtained and purified from pork and beef and is also available as pure human insulin from recombinant DNA technology. Insulins can be long or short acting. Regular insulin is short-acting while NPH insulin has activity for a longer period. These are the two most common types of insulin in use today. Also available are mixtures of regular and NPH insulins which may be easier for diabetics to use. Some of the common brand names of insulin are listed below:

- Humulin®
- Mixtard®
- Iletin®
- Novolin®

Uses

Blood sugars must be tested several times daily as levels of activity and stress as well as illness affect blood sugar. Patients may give supplemental doses of insulin if the blood sugar is too high. All insulins other than regular are suspensions and should be gently swirled before use to disperse the insulin crystals.

The ranking of insulin types from fastest onset of action to slowest is as follows: Regular, NPH, Lente, Ultralente. The faster an insulin exerts its effect, the greater that effect is. However, the faster-acting insulins also are cleared from the body more rapidly, and the more injections of that insulin must be given daily to control the blood sugar.

Dosage Forms

Regular insulin is the only type of insulin which may be given intravenously; all other types may have very serious side effects when given intravenously. Insulin may be given only subcutaneously or intravenously and must be administered daily for the rest of a person's life.

✤ SIDE EFFECTS:

Insulin must be dosed individually for each person to avoid giving either too little or too much as either may produce negative side effects. **Too little insulin** may cause increased blood sugar that may result in coma. **Too much insulin** may cause dizziness and lead to coma because the brain needs sugar in the blood in order to function. Blood sugars must be tested several times daily as levels of activity and stress as well as illness affects blood sugar. Patients may give supplemental doses of insulin if the blood sugar is too high.

Sulfonylureas

Persons who produce small quantities of insulin may not need insulin. The sulfonylureas stimulate the pancreas to release more insulin. Some common oral sulfonylureas are listed below:

GENERIC	TRADE
• acetohexamide	• Dymelor®
• chlorpropamide	• Diabinese®
• glipizide	• Glucotrol®
• glyburide	• Micronase®
• tolazamide	• Tolinase®
• tolbutamide	• Orinase®

Uses

The sulfonylureas are not hormones, but they do stimulate the secretion of the hormone insulin. In addition, these drugs make the cells more sensitive to the actions of insulin.

The earliest developed sulfonylureas (chlorpropamide, acetohexamide) cause patients to have greater problems with hypoglycemia (low blood sugar) than the newest agents (glyburide, glipizide).

Unlike insulin, larger doses of these drugs have an increased effect only up to a certain point. If a patient does not completely respond to maximum doses of these drugs, insulin may be added for additional control.

Dosage Forms

The sulfonylureas are available only in oral forms.

✤ SIDE EFFECTS:

Stomach upset; these drugs also interact with alcohol to cause flushing, nausea and headache.

Thyroid Hormone

The thyroid is a small gland in the neck that produces thyroid hormones important for metabolism. Some of the natural and synthetic thyroid hormones are listed below:

GENERIC	TRADE
levothyroxine sodium	Synthroid®, Levothroid®
liothyronine sodium	Cytomel®
liotrix	Thyrolar®, Euthroid®
thyroglobulin	Proloid®
thyroid	Armour Thyroid®

Uses

The thyroid hormones regulate many aspects of metabolism; including carbohydrate metabolism and muscle construction and destruction. Without these hormones, the body cannot efficiently carry out its metabolic functions.

The most commonly used thyroid hormone is levothyroxine (Synthroid®), a synthetic compound. Some of the products on the market are formed from freeze-dried animal thyroid gland. The effect from these products is harder to predict than from the synthetic hormones.

Dosage Forms

All of the above products are available in tablet form. Additionally, thyroid is available as coated tablets and capsules. Only levothyroxine is available in an injectable form.

✤ SIDE EFFECTS:

These hormones must be administered in the proper dose. **Too little thyroid hormone** will cause sluggishness, depression, weight gain and cold intolerance. **Too much thyroid hormone** will cause irritability, nervousness, weight loss, and heat intolerance.

Local Anesthetic Agents

The local anesthetics are agents used to produce numbness in certain areas or to deaden pain. These agents may be injected or applied topically to the necessary area. Some of the local anesthetic agents are listed below:

GENERIC	TRADE
benzocaine	Oracin, Oratect
bupivacaine HCl	Marcaine HCl®
chloroprocaine	Nesacaine®
cocaine	
etidocaine	Duranest HCl®
lidocaine	Xylocaine®

44 *Basic Pharmacology*

GENERIC	TRADE
• mepivacaine HCl	• Carbocaine®
• procaine	• Novocain®
• tetracaine	• Pontocaine®

Uses

Local anesthetics work by blocking the movement of sodium into and out of nerve cells. By blocking this movement, local anesthetics prevent the generation of a nerve impulse.

Local anesthetics are sometimes injected into the area around the spinal cord to block pain signals during surgery. When used in this manner, a preparation must be used which does not contain any preservatives to avoid possible spinal cord damage.

Lidocaine is also often given intravenously to control arrhythmias. The mechanism of lidocaine's action on the heart is the same as that responsible for its numbing ability—the blockade of sodium movement into and out of cells.

Dosage Forms

All of the above except benzocaine and tetracaine are injectable drugs. Benzocaine is available in creams, lotions, ointments, solutions, lozenges, topical aerosols, and gels. Tetracaine is available in solutions, sprays, liquids, ointments, and gels.

✣ SIDE EFFECTS:

Burning (when injected or applied to skin or mucous membranes); heart arrhythmias (if too much is given or if the drug gets into the bloodstream).

MUSCLE RELAXANTS

There are several groups of muscle relaxants. The smooth muscle relaxants are used for disorders of the bladder and respiratory system. The skeletal muscle relaxants are used to treat muscle spasms.

Bladder Muscle Relaxants

The smooth muscle relaxants used for the bladder work by decreasing bladder spasms. Some common bladder smooth muscle relaxants are listed below:

GENERIC	TRADE
• flavoxate HCl	• Urispas®
• oxybutynin chloride	• Ditropan®

Uses

Smooth muscle relaxants are used to decrease bladder spasms which can cause frequency or urgency of urination and may lead to incontinence.

Dosage Forms

Flavoxate is available as tablets only; oxybutynin is available in solution and tablet form.

✥ SIDE EFFECTS:

Dry mouth; decreased sweating; flushing; rapid heartbeat; blurred vision

Respiratory Smooth Muscle Relaxants

The respiratory smooth muscle relaxants work by directly relaxing the smooth muscles of the trachea or windpipe and the bronchi in the lung allowing easier breathing. Some common respiratory smooth muscle relaxants are listed below:

GENERIC	TRADE
• aminophylline	• Phyllocontin®
• dyphylline	• Dilor®
• oxtriphylline	• Choledyl®
• theophylline	• Theo-Dur®, Slo-Phyllin®, Slo-Bid®

Uses

Theophylline and aminophylline are used most commonly in practice. Aminophylline is converted to theophylline in the body. It is 80% as potent as theophylline on a milligram-for-milligram basis. Therefore, 100 mg of aminophylline has the same potency as 80 mg of theophylline. It was once thought that the mechanism of theophylline's action was understood, but it is now known that the true mechanism has not been proven. It seems that the more we learn, the less we actually know about this drug.

When a patient presents with a severe asthma attack, theophylline is started as a continuous infusion after a loading dose generally in combination with a steroidal anti-inflammatory such as methylprednisolone. Theophylline blood levels must be closely monitored as many drugs interact with theophylline, and toxic symptoms can be severe. The lowest rate of infusion that will control symptoms should be used to prevent toxicity.

Oral theophylline is used on patients who have had their disease stabilized. The sustained release dosage forms are used commonly because they are more convenient for patients to take.

Oxtriphylline is 64% as potent as theophylline and is converted to theophylline by the body. Dyphylline is a derivative of theophylline but is not converted to theophylline. It may have fewer side effects than theophylline but is less potent.

Dosage Forms

Theophylline is available as an injectable and as tablets, capsules, elixir, solutions, and liquids. The sustained-release forms should not be crushed or chewed to prevent release of a large amount of drug at one time, which could lead to toxicity. Aminophylline is available in tablet, rectal suppository, rectal solution, elixir, oral liquid, tablet, and injectable forms. Dyphylline is available in tablet, elixir and injectable forms.

✥ SIDE EFFECTS:

Arrhythmias, stomach upset, rapid heartbeat, irritability, nervousness and seizures. **Note:** The amount of drug necessary for effective activity is very close to the amount of drug that leads to toxicity. The concentrations of these drugs in the patient's blood should be monitored regularly.

Skeletal Muscle Relaxants

The skeletal muscle relaxants are used to treat mild to severe muscle spasms. Some of the skeletal muscle relaxants are listed below:

GENERIC	TRADE
baclofen	Lioresal®
carisoprodol	Soma®
chlorzoxazone	Parafon Forte®
dantrolene sodium	Dantrium®
methocarbamol	Robaxin®
orphenadrine citrate	Norflex®
cyclobenzrapine HCl	Flexiril®

Uses

Of the above list, only dantrolene directly relaxes the skeletal muscle; the other drugs act within the brain stem or spinal cord to abort muscle spasms. Dantrolene is used in the treatment of **malignant hyperthermia**, a condition occasionally triggered by general anesthesia and frequently observed in massive cocaine overdoses. In this condition, muscular metabolic and contractile ability increase to such an extent that the heat produced becomes life-threatening. Because dantrolene directly causes muscle relaxation, the drug can treat this condition quickly. Baclofen is primarily used to treat muscle spasms associated with multiple sclerosis. The remaining agents are used to treat muscle spasms associated with muscular injury, primarily back strain. Diazepam (Valium®) is widely used in the treatment of muscle spasms also. It appears that it is effective because of its effects both at the area of the spinal cord and at the brain stem.

Dosage Forms

Baclofen may be given orally or injected intrathecally (into the area around the spinal cord.) Likewise, dantrolene, methocarbamol and orphenadrine are available in tablet and injectable forms. Carisoprodol and chlorzoxazone are available in tablet form only.

✣ SIDE EFFECTS:

Dizziness, weakness, drowsiness, nausea

Neuromuscular-blocking agents

The neuromuscular blockers are utilized when complete paralysis is necessary. Most often these drugs are used when the patient requires a machine to breathe for him or her (mechanical ventilation). Paralysis is needed in this instance because many patients will try to fight the ventilator and injure themselves in the process. Some of the neuromuscular blockers are listed below:

GENERIC	TRADE
atracurium besylate	Tracrium®
pancuronium bromide	Pavulon®
succinylcholine	Anectine®
vecuronium bromide	Norcuron®

The first neuromuscular blocker discovered was curare—a drug which occurs naturally in a plant in South America. This is the substance responsible for the effects of "poison-tipped arrows" which are referred to in many stories. While the effects of these arrows were much exaggerated, the drug did create a major breakthrough for medical science. Use of curare allowed surgeons to operate on a patient who would lie perfectly still, thus increasing the precision of delicate operations and allowing procedures to be performed which were previously impossible.

Neuromuscular blocking agents may be given in small, frequent doses or as a continuous infusion. To prevent an overdose of these medications, health care workers make use of a peripheral nerve stimulator—an electrical device which can deliver a small shock to a muscle. When the muscle is shocked, it should twitch 1-3 times before relaxing again. If no twitches occur, too much drug is being given. If more than 3 twitches occur, then not enough drug is being given.

Dosage Forms

All of the above drugs are injectable or infusible.

✢ SIDE EFFECTS:

Drowsiness, stomach upset, nausea, dry mouth, dizziness

VITAMINS

Vitamins are natural substances found in food that are necessary for many cellular functions in the body. There are two main groups of vitamins—the water-soluble vitamins which are absorbed into the body, used, and excreted and the fat-soluble vitamins which are absorbed into the body and stored.

Water-Soluble Vitamins

Common water-soluble vitamins include:

GENERIC	TRADE
ascorbic acid	Vitamin C
cyanocobalamin	Vitamin B_{12}
folate or folic acid	Vitamin B_9
niacin or nicotinic acid	Vitamin B_3
pantothenic acid	
pyridoxine	Vitamin B_6
riboflavin	Vitamin B_2
thiamine	Vitamin B_1

Fat-Soluble Vitamins

Common fat-soluble vitamins include:

GENERIC	TRADE
beta carotene	Vitamin A
calcifediol, calcitriol, dihydrotachysterol, ergocalciferol	Vitamin D

GENERIC	TRADE
• calciferol	• Vitamin E
• menadione, phytonadione	• Vitamin K

Many claims are made about the ability of vitamins to prevent or cure disease. Most of these claims are false. However, some are true or are presently being studied.

Folic acid appears to be responsible for development of a healthy spinal cord in the fetus. Supplementation is presently recommended for women who desire to become or are presently pregnant.

The antioxidant vitamins (Vitamin C, Vitamin E, and beta carotene) are presently being studied to determine their role in the prevention of cardiovascular disease. The results of some studies support supplementation, while others do not. Vitamin C has also been demonstrated to be needed in larger amounts in critically ill patients; especially those patients with unhealed wounds.

Vitamin K is responsible for the formation of blood clotting factors. Persons taking the anticoagulant warfarin need to maintain a consistent level of this vitamin in their body for the drug to have a predictable effect on blood coagulation time.

The primary effect of Vitamin D is to increase calcium absorption from the intestine. It is used in the treatment of hypocalcemia (low blood calcium levels), hypophosphatemia (low blood phosphorous levels), and rickets.

Folic acid and thiamine are given to alcoholics upon admission to a hospital. Alcoholics typically have poor diets and may not get enough of these vitamins. A thiamine deficiency can cause confusion, hallucinations, abnormal carbohydrate metabolism, coma and death (Wernicke-Korsakoff syndrome).

Dosage Forms

The vitamins are available in numerous forms, including, but certainly not limited to, tablets, powders, capsules, liquids and injectable forms.

✣ SIDE EFFECTS:

Vitamins are generally considered non toxic, but the fat-soluble vitamins can accumulate if too many are taken. This accumulation may lead to nausea, vomiting and some liver abnormalities. Most vitamins are available as multivitamin products that contain at least the amount suggested for the Recommended Dietary Allowance (RDA). Vitamin supplementation is generally not necessary in healthy persons because the normal diet will provide the amount necessary for the body to function properly.

UNIT II

Preparation and Handling of Sterile products

Chapter 4
PHARMACY-PREPARED STERILE PRODUCTS

In this chapter:
- *Routes of Administration*
- *Types of Solution Systems*
- *Methods of Administration*

SCOPE OF PRACTICE

The preparation of sterile products has become an increasingly important aspect of pharmacy practice. Changes in the health care environment, new drug products, and advancing technology have all contributed to the need for these services in hospitals and expansion into the home health care setting.

Points to Remember

- The extent of pharmacy-prepared sterile products programs varies not only from institution to institution but from practice setting to practice setting.
- All of these programs have a common goal of providing accurately prepared sterile products for administration to patients.
- The pharmacy technician is an integral part in the preparation of these sterile products.

ROUTES OF ADMINISTRATION

There are many routes by which sterile products may be administered. The route chosen will depend on the intended site of action, the desired effect of the medication and the characteristics of the medication to be administered. The following describes some of the different routes of administration.

- *Intradermal (I.D.):* Injection just below the skin surface; usually used for diagnostic tests and some vaccines. Total volume does not exceed 0.1 ml.
- *Subcutaneous (S.C.):* Injection deeper than I.D. into the loose tissue beneath the skin. Total volume does not exceed 1 ml.
- *Intramuscular (I.M.):* Injection into a muscle mass. A common site is the deltoid muscle of the upper arm, into which a maximum of 2 ml may be injected. Volumes up to 5 ml may be injected into the gluteal muscle of the buttocks.
- *Intravenous (I.V.):* Large or small volumes of solutions are injected directly into the veins.
- *Intra-arterial (I.A.):* Medications are injected directly into an artery. This is used to administer medication (i.e., radiopaque, certain antineoplastic agents) directly to a target organ.
- *Intrathecal (I.T.):* Medications are injected directly into the spinal fluid. Preservative-free medications must be used as many preservatives can damage the nervous system.
- *Topical:* Application of the medication to the surface site of action. This is used for medications such as irrigations, eye drops and ear drops.

Types of Solution Systems

Intravenous solutions are usually classified as small volume parenterals (SVP) or large volume parenterals (LVP). SVPs are usually 100 ml or less and are used as vehicles for delivery of medications. LVPs are solutions of more than 100 ml and are generally used to correct fluid, electrolyte and/or nutrient imbalances but may also be used as vehicles for medication delivery.

There are four types of solution systems, or containers, currently used in the preparation of sterile products:

- Glass containers with air tube
- Glass containers without air tube
- Flexible plastic containers
- Semi-rigid plastic containers

Both types of glass containers are packed under a vacuum and sealed with a rubber closure, or diaphragm, held in place by an aluminum band. In order for the solution to flow out of a glass container, air must be able to enter the container as solution flows out. This is accomplished through an air tube or through a vented administration set.

Flexible plastic containers are the most common solution system. They are lightweight and unbreakable. At the top of the container is a flat plastic extension with a hole to allow the container to be hung from the administration pole. At the opposite end of the container are two ports—one for adding medication to the solution and the other as the entry port for the administration set.

Semi-rigid plastic containers are frequently used for irrigation solutions. These solutions are used to rinse open wounds or body cavities and are only used topically, never by injection.

METHODS OF ADMINISTRATION

Sterile products may be administered to the patient in one of several ways:

- Injection
- I.V. push
- I.V. (continuous) infusion

- Intermittent (piggyback) infusion,
- Irrigation

Injection involves the administration of a small volume of medication by means of a needle and syringe by one of the following routes: intradermal (I.D.), subcutaneous (S.C.), intramuscular (I.M.), intra-arterial (I.A.), or intrathecal (I.T.).

I.V. push involves the injection of a small volume of medication by means of a needle and syringe over a short period of time. This involves administration of the medication directly into a vein or into the tubing of a running I.V. solution. This method is used when a very rapid effect is desired and is sometimes referred to as a bolus.

I.V. infusion, or continuous infusion, involves the administration of large amounts of solution directly into the vein over a relatively long period of time. Infusions are used to correct fluid and/or electrolyte imbalances and as a vehicle for medications and nutrients.

Intermittent, or piggyback, infusions are used to deliver medications in small volumes of fluid (usually 50 - 100 ml) into the tubing of a flowing I.V. solution (primary I.V.). The solution is administered over a short time period (30 - 60 minutes) at specified intervals. The solution is contained in a minibag or bottle. A variation of the piggyback infusion method involves the use of syringes instead of the piggyback containers to deliver the medication to the patient. The syringe is connected to a syringe pump which delivers the contents of the syringe over a specific period of time.

Irrigation solutions are not to be administered by injection. These solutions are generally used topically to flush open wounds.

I.V. solutions flow from the container to the patient by means of an administration set. These sets have at one end a spike which is inserted into the stopper site of the rubber closure of the solution container. The solution flows from the inverted solution container into a drip chamber and through a length of tubing which has a Leur-lock needle adapter at the other end. A roller clamp on the tubing provides regulation of the flow rate.

Chapter 5
ASEPTIC TECHNIQUE AND STERILE PRODUCT PREPARATION

In this chapter:
- *Theory of Aseptic Technique*
- *Laminar Airflow Hoods*
- *Types of Airflow Hoods*
- *General Principles for Operation*

THEORY OF ASEPTIC TECHNIQUE

The majority of sterile products involve injectable medications which may be administered to patients by several techniques and for many reasons. It is important to remember that injectable medications bypass important barriers to infection (i.e., skin, gastric mucosa). Bacteria exist everywhere. The introduction of bacteria into a patient can be limited by assuring that the medications which are to be administered to the patient are not contaminated with bacteria. These contaminants may be introduced from the environment, equipment, devices, or personnel. Therefore, all objects that come into contact with an injectable, an I.V. solution, or an irrigation, must be sterile or contamination will result.

Points to Remember
- Aseptic technique is defined as the procedures utilized to prevent bacterial contamination during the preparation of a sterile product.
- This technique involves control of the environment and procedures used in product preparation.

LAMINAR AIRFLOW HOODS

Contamination can occur from the environment in which the product is prepared and from the person preparing the product. Room air contains thousands of suspended particles per cubic foot such as dust, pollens, and bacteria. These contaminants must be reduced in order to provide a clean environment for sterile product preparation.

There are several steps that can be taken to minimize the number of particulates in the air. The sterile compounding area should be cleaned daily and be separated from routine pharmacy operations, nonessential equipment, and other material, such as cardboard boxes, that produce particles. Traffic flow into the sterile compounding area should also be minimized.

An effective way to significantly minimize external particulate contamination from entering the sterile compounding area is to prepare sterile products in a laminar airflow hood. However, the use of poor aseptic technique will negatively impact on the benefits of the laminar airflow hood.

The use of a laminar airflow hood creates a "Class 100" environment for the preparation of sterile products. This means that the airflow within the hood contains no more than 100 particles per cubic foot that are 0.5 microns or larger in size. The laminar airflow hood filters and suspends any particulate contamination that is introduced into the airflow through the hood by means of straight parallel air streams. This process creates an environment in which aseptic procedures can be correctly performed.

Types of Laminar Airflow Hoods

There are two types of laminar airflow hoods—horizontal and vertical flow. Horizontal flow hoods are used for the preparation of the majority of sterile products. This type of hood initially draws contaminated room air through a prefilter by means of the hood's electric blower (see **Figure 1**).

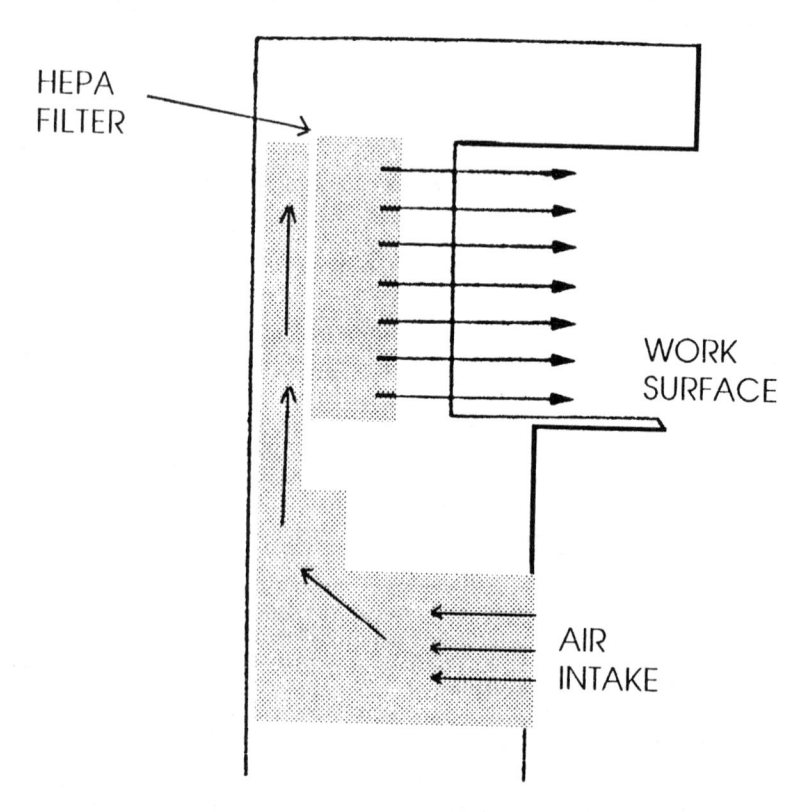

Figure 1: Horizontal Laminar Air Flow Hood

The prefilter removes large size particulates and must be replaced on a regular basis, just as with a furnace filter. The prefiltered air is then pressurized and moved to the high-efficiency particulate air (HEPA) filter, which comprises the entire back portion of the hood's work area. The HEPA filter removes 99.97% of all particles larger than 0.3 microns in size which essentially includes all airborne microorganisms and particulate matter. The filtered air flows horizontally at a constant, high velocity sufficient to keep the work area free from contaminated room air.

Vertical flow hoods, or biological safety cabinets (BSCs), are used for the preparation of hazardous drugs, such as antineoplastic (anticancer) drugs. Class II BSCs create a vertical flow air barrier, or curtain, between you and the work area, protecting you from hazardous drug particles generated during sterile product preparation (See **Figures 2** on page 56 and **Figure 3** on page 57). Additionally, the front glass shield must always be properly positioned for protection and to maintain the vertical airflow. These hoods draw contaminated room air in through the front intake grate and filter it through a HEPA filter. The filtered air then passes vertically downward through the work area and is drawn out the front intake grate and rear exhaust grate. It is important to remember that objects should not be placed on or near the front intake or rear exhaust grates as this will obstruct the airflow and reduce the effectiveness of the BSC.

There are two important types of Class II BSCs. Type A BSCs pump 30% of the air filtered by the HEPA filter back into the room air (**Figure 2**). The exhaust filter must not be blocked. Type B BSCs pump air from the work zone through a HEPA filter and exhausts this filtered air to the outside of the building through an auxiliary exhaust system (Figure 3). This exhaust mechanism also promotes a faster inward flow of air. Type B BSCs, therefore, offer greater protection and are preferred over Type A BSCs for the preparation of hazardous drugs.

The most important factor in utilizing laminar airflow hoods is that no object is to interrupt the flow of air between the HEPA filter and a sterile object. Any foreign object (bottles, hands, etc.) placed between a sterile object and the HEPA filter provides an opportunity for contaminants from the foreign object to be carried by the air currents to the sterile object ..Therefore, in order to eliminate the contamination risk, no object should pass behind a sterile object in a horizontal flow hood nor above a sterile object in a vertical flow hood.

Additionally, all objects placed in the work area of the hood are to be placed in a manner that will allow maximum efficiency of the airflow at all times. Objects placed at the back of the work area next to the HEPA filter, against a vertical wall, or within 6 inches from the front of the hood, create an extended area of turbulence behind the object. This turbulence allows contaminated air to exist or to be pulled into the hood.

General Principles for Operation

There are some general principles that should be followed for the proper operation of laminar airflow hoods:

- Hoods should be positioned in a controlled area away from excess traffic, doors, air vents, etc. that may cause air currents capable of allowing contaminants to enter the work area.
- Before use, all interior work surfaces of the hood should be cleaned (see "Cleaning and Maintenance").
- All aseptic manipulations should occur at least 6 inches inside of the hood to prevent turbulence that may pull contaminated air into the work area. To achieve this, work with your arms extended into the work area so that your elbows are away from your sides.
- Nothing should come in contact with the HEPA filter.
- Jewelry should not be worn on the hands or wrists when working in the hood as this may introduce particles or bacteria into the work area.

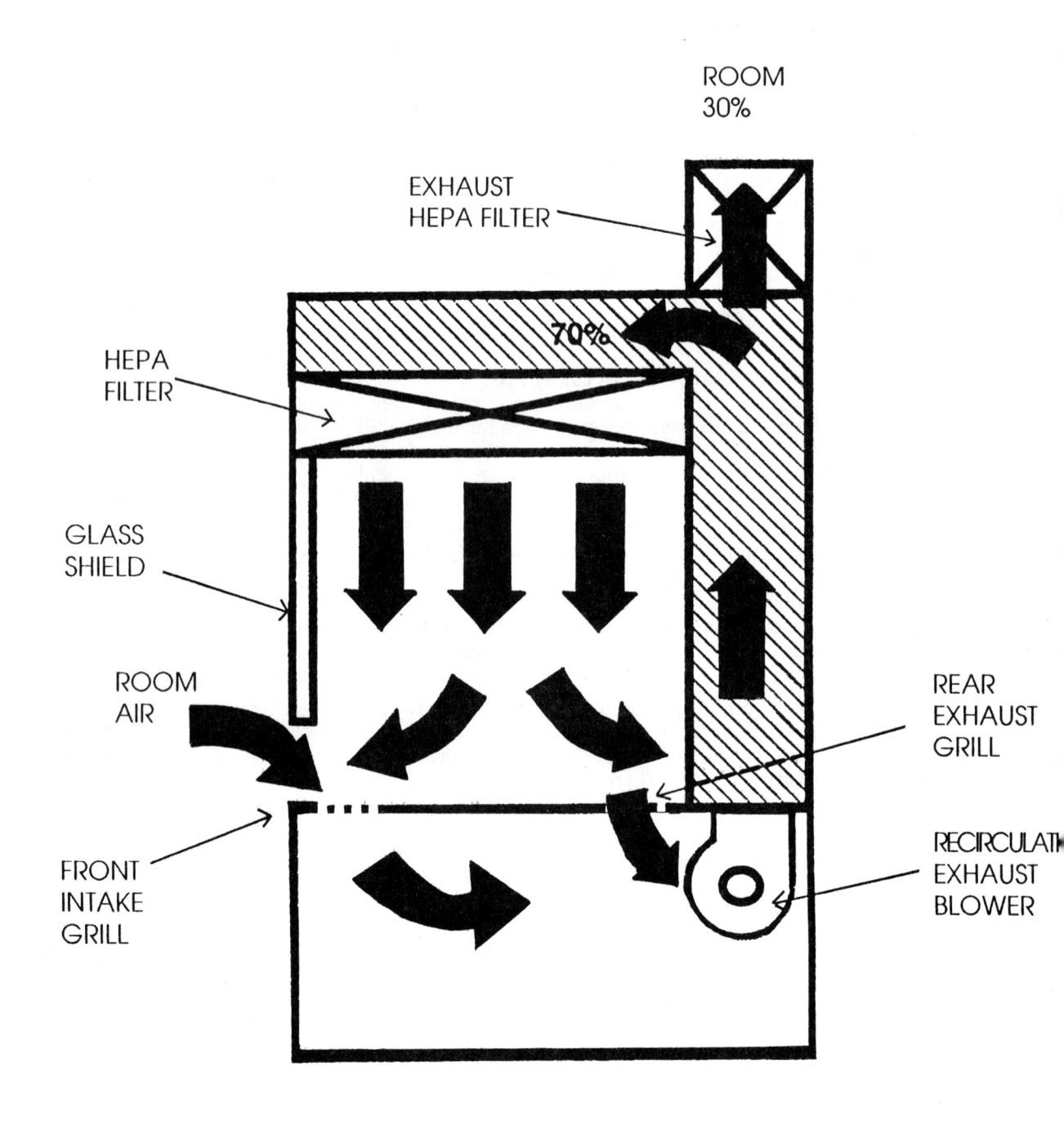

Figure 2: Class II Type A Biological Safety Cabinet

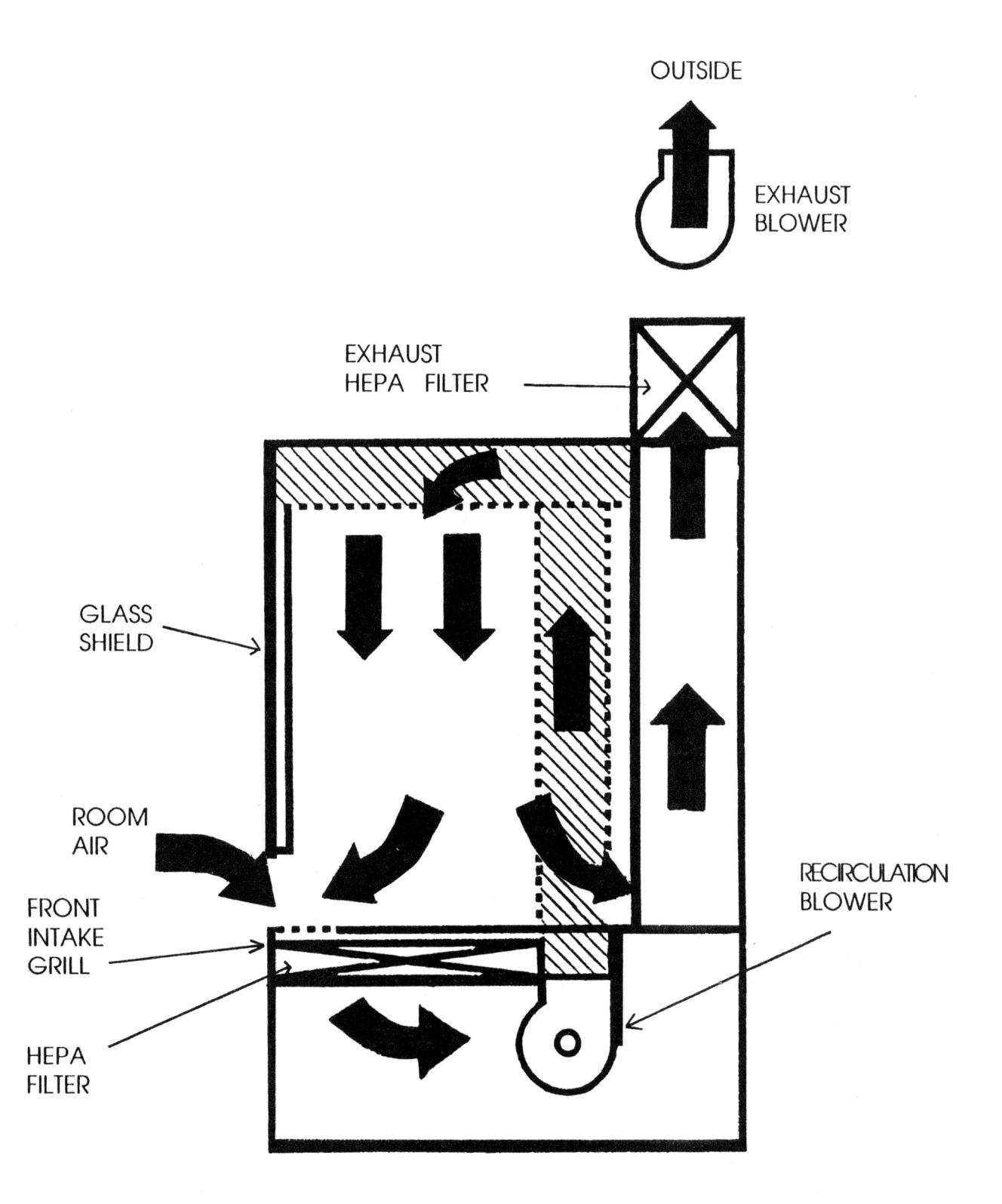

Figure 3: Class II Type B Biological Safety Cabinet

- Talking, sneezing and coughing should be directed away from the hood work area to minimize turbulence of the airflow.
- Only those objects essential to preparation of the sterile product should be properly placed in the work area. Items such as paper, pens, labels or supply trays are not to be placed in the hood.
- Laminar airflow hoods are designed to operate continuously. If a horizontal airflow hood is turned off between sterile product preparations, it is recommended that the hood operate at least 30 minutes to allow complete removal of room air from the work area, then disinfected before use. Vertical airflow hoods must be operated continuously, 24 hours a day to prevent contamination of room air.
- The number of people working in a laminar airflow hood should be minimized in order to reduce turbulence of airflow.

Remember: Although the laminar airflow hood creates a clean environment for the aseptic manipulation of sterile products, the hood alone, without the strict observance of aseptic technique, will not insure a sterile product.

Cleaning and Maintenance

All laminar airflow hoods must have a regular schedule for cleaning and maintenance.

- All hood work areas and all interior surfaces are to be cleaned with 70% isopropyl alcohol or other appropriate disinfectant before each use and periodically throughout the sterile preparation process. Horizontal airflow hoods should be cleaned and disinfected from back to front, away from the HEPA filter. Plexiglass side panels should be cleaned with a warm, soapy water solution, as alcohol may damage the panels.
- Biological safety cabinets (BSCs) should have the back and side panels cleaned and disinfected before each use and periodically throughout the sterile preparation process. Cleaning and disinfection should occur in the direction of the vertical airflow, starting with the top and working down towards the work area.
- Additionally, BSCs should be decontaminated weekly or in the event of a large spill. Special considerations are required for this procedure:
  - You must wear a gown, latex gloves covered by utility gloves, hair cover and eye protection (the glass shield may need to be raised). The blower is to remain on during the decontamination. Clean back and side panels from top to bottom, using heavy toweling or gauze with a cleaner and distilled water. The cover to the HEPA filter is removed and cleaned. The work tray should be lifted and leaned against the back wall and cleaned underneath. The spill trough and drain should be thoroughly scrubbed. Discard cleaner and water containers as contaminated waste along with all protective apparel and cleaning materials.
  - Exterior surfaces of the hood, as well as all other active work surfaces in the controlled area, should be regularly disinfected.
  - Prefilters should be changed periodically.
  - Hoods are to be inspected and certified by qualified personnel at least every 6 months, whenever the hood is moved, or if damage to the HEPA filter is suspected. This ensures the operational efficiency and integrity of the hood.

Chapter 6
PERSONNEL

In this chapter:
- *Education, Training and Evaluation*
- *Attire*
- *Handwashing*
- *Supplies*

EDUCATION, TRAINING AND EVALUATION

Personnel preparing sterile products should receive appropriate lecture and experiential training and competency evaluation by demonstration and/or testing (written or practical) of the preparation of sterile products. Personnel should be knowledgeable with respect to aseptic technique and preparation procedures, appropriate attire, controlled area contamination factors, equipment, supplies, calculations and terminology.

Points to Remember:

- Aseptic technique for each person preparing sterile products should be observed and evaluated, including written or practical tests, on a regular basis.
- This should occur during orientation and training and at regular intervals thereafter.
- Most practice settings perform this function at least annually, with 6 months becoming the usual interval for evaluation.

Once aseptic technique is observed and evaluated, the process should be validated through process simulation to assure consistency in the quality of sterile products. Process simulation testing allows for evaluation of bacterial contamination during each step of the sterile product preparation process. The testing is performed in the same manner as normal preparation, except that bacterial growth medium is utilized in the process as if it were the product to be prepared for a patient. The medium samples are then incubated and evaluated for bacterial growth; no growth indicates that adequate aseptic technique was utilized, while bacterial growth indicates improper aseptic technique. When bacterial growth is evident, the complete preparation process must be re-evaluated, appropriate corrective actions taken, and process simulation testing repeated.

Attire

Personnel attire is the first component of good aseptic technique. Specific attire may vary according to practice setting; however, personnel should generally wear clean clothing covers that are particle free when working in the controlled area. Clothing covers should have a closed front and long sleeves with elastic cuffs. Jewelry on the hands or wrists should be minimized, and preferably eliminated, to reduce bacterial and particulate contamination. Masks and gloves (nonpowdered) are recommended and head and facial hair should be covered. Shoe covers may also be useful in reducing bacterial and particulate contamination.

Handwashing

The laminar airflow hood, if used appropriately, eliminates almost all airborne contaminants. Therefore, touch contamination is the most common route by which a sterile product may become contaminated. Your hands contain numerous bacterial and particulate contaminants, and proper handwashing becomes extremely important in eliminating sterile product contamination.

Personnel preparing sterile products should thoroughly scrub hands, nails, wrists and forearms (to the elbow). A brush, warm water, and an appropriate bactericidal soap, such as chlorhexidine, should be employed for at least a 30 second period. Handwashing must occur prior to wearing gloves and should be performed frequently, especially after leaving and returning to the controlled area.

It is important to emphasize that gloves do not remain sterile during the preparation process. Gloves should be rinsed frequently with 70% isopropyl alcohol, or other compatible disinfectant, and changed whenever their integrity is compromised.

Supplies

Another important factor in the aseptic preparation of sterile products is the correct use of supplies, such as syringes and needles. Syringes and needles are used for almost all sterile product preparation.

Syringes are classified according to their composition: glass (reusable, disposable) or plastic (disposable). Glass syringes, which are used primarily for medications requiring glass for stability or storage purposes, are costly and are, therefore, infrequently used. Disposable plastic syringes are most frequently used, as they are less expensive and stability problems are minimal during the short period of time the medication is in contact with the plastic.

Syringes are available in sizes from 1 ml to 60 ml capacity and all have the same basic structure: They are equipped with a plunger inside a barrel (See **Figure 4** on page 61). The plunger passes inside the barrel of the syringe and has a flat disc for manipulation outside of the barrel and a cone-shaped rubber piston at the end inside the barrel. The barrel is graduated in milliliters—smaller increments and a long slender barrel for accuracy with small volume syringes and larger increments for larger syringes. To measure with a syringe, line up the edge of the plunger piston closest to the tip in contact with the barrel with the graduation increment on the barrel that corresponds to the volume desired. The collar of the syringe is utilized to prevent the syringe from slipping during aseptic manipulation. The tip is the point of attachment for the needle. Most syringes have a locking mechanism (Leurlock) at the tip. This mechanism secures the needle within a threaded ring and prevents the needle from slipping off of the tip. Some syringes do not have this locking mechanism; instead the needle is held on the syringe tip by friction.

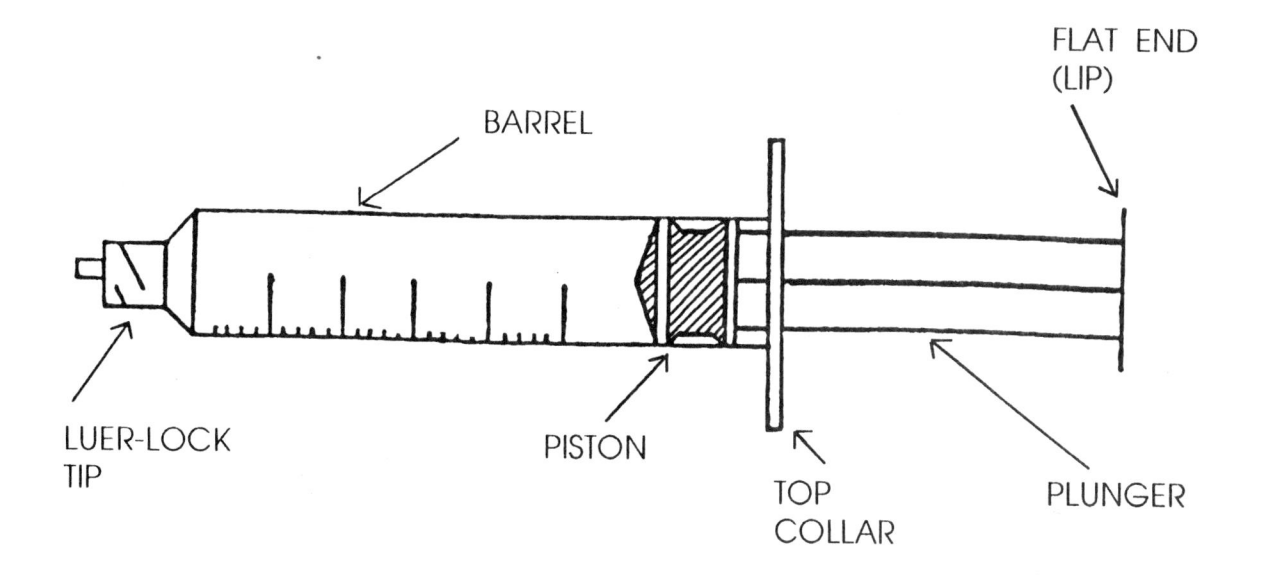

Figure 4: Luer-Lock Syringe

Syringes are individually packaged by the manufacturer in sterile overwraps. The sterility of the syringe is guaranteed as long as the overwrap is intact. The intact package should be opened only within the laminar airflow hood in order to maintain this sterility. If the integrity of the package is broken before placement in the laminar airflow hood, the syringe should be discarded.

Syringes are usually packaged with a protective cover over the syringe tip. This protector should be left in place until it is time to attach the needle. Attachment of needles to syringes with a Leur-lock tip requires a quarter-turn to secure the needle to the syringe. Non-Leur-lock tips rely on friction to hold the needle on the syringe tip.

Needles, like syringes, are available in many sizes. Needle size is designated by two numbers indicating gauge and length. The gauge of the needle corresponds to the needle's bore. Needle gauge ranges from 28, the finest, to 13, the thickest or largest. The length of the needle represents the length of the shaft in inches and usually ranges from ⅜ to 3 ½ inches.

Needles consist of two parts: the hub and the shaft (See **Figure 5** on page 62). The hub is used to attach the needle to the syringe and may be color-coded to correspond to a specific gauge size. The tip of the needle shaft is slanted to form a point. The slant of the point is called the bevel, the point is called the bevel tip and the opposite end of the slant is designated the bevel heel.

Like syringes, needles are individually packaged by the manufacturer in sterile overwraps. The sterility of the needle is guaranteed as long as the overwrap is intact; the intact package should be opened only in the laminar airflow hood in order to maintain this sterility. If the integrity of the package is broken before placement in the laminar airflow hood, the needle should be discarded.

62 *Personnel*

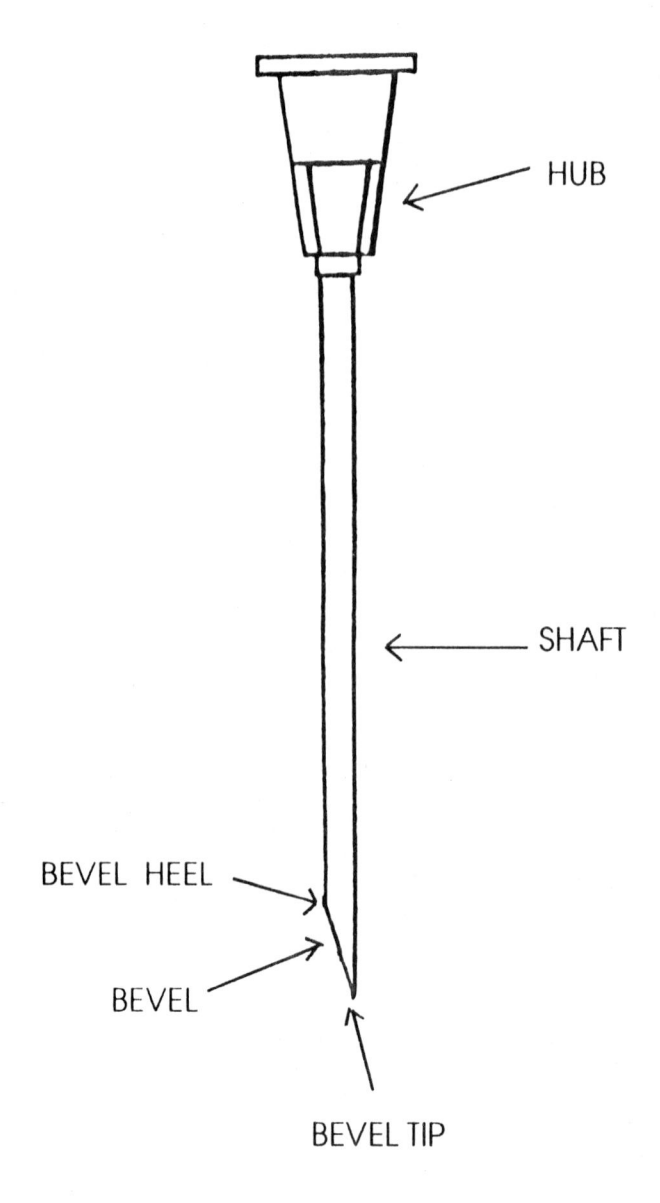

- HUB
- SHAFT
- BEVEL HEEL
- BEVEL
- BEVEL TIP

Figure 5: Needle

The needle shaft is usually metal and lubricated with a sterile silicone coating; should not be swabbed with alcohol. No part of a needle should be touched. All manipulation of a needle should occur by the protective cover only. When attaching the needle to the syringe tip, keep fingers well away from the point of attachment of the syringe to the needle. The protective cover is left in place until the needle and syringe are to be used for an aseptic manipulation.

Chapter 7
PROPER HANDLING OF STERILE PRODUCTS

In this chapter:
- *Manipulation of Contents of a Vial*
- *Manipulation of Contents of an Ampule*
- *Medication Transfers*
- *Inspecting Final Sterile Product*
- *Antineoplastic Medications*

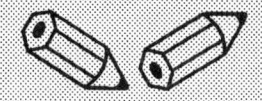

MANIPULATION OF CONTENTS OF A VIAL

A vial is a glass container with a rubber stopper secured to its top by an aluminum band. The following steps make possible the aseptic removal of the liquid contents of a vial utilizing a syringe and needle:

- Remove the protective outer tab and swab the top of the rubber stopper of the vial with 70% isopropyl alcohol. The alcohol is required as the protective cap does not guarantee sterility. Swabbing should occur with several firm strokes in the same direction over the rubber stopper. This disinfects and removes particles from the rubber stopper.

- Vials are a closed system. To prevent a vacuum from forming in the vial, air must replace the volume of fluid that is to be removed. Pull the needle protective cover straight off. Next, pull out the plunger to the volume you wish to remove. This equals the amount of air to inject into the vial prior to withdrawing the liquid.

- Place the needle on the surface of the rubber stopper so that the bevel side faces upward. It is important to prevent "coring" the rubber stopper when inserting the needle. (Cores are pieces of the rubber stopper carved out when the needle is inserted into the vial.) To prevent "coring", first begin piercing the rubber stopper with the bevel tip and then apply lateral (towards the bevel) and downward pressure on the syringe to insert the needle at an angle of 45°.

- Push the needle so the beveled tip is well into the vial and inject the volume of air.
- Invert the syringe and the vial so that one hand holds the vial and the other hand the barrel of the syringe.
- The needle should be positioned to just penetrate the rubber closure to allow all the medication to be withdrawn, if needed. Use the thumb to pull back the plunger without touching the plunger barrel.
- After withdrawing the volume needed, tap the syringe to move any air bubbles to the needle end.
- Expel any air and excess volume prior to removing needle from vial.
- Cap the needle when done.

MANIPULATION OF CONTENTS OF AN AMPULE

An ampule is a small glass container of medication solution that must be broken to remove the liquid. A colored ring is often found on the ampule neck indicating the weak point at which the ampule is to be broken. The following steps allow for the aseptic removal of the contents of an ampule utilizing a syringe and needle.

- Hold the ampule upright, and tap the top to remove any liquid trapped in this area.
- Swab the neck of the ampule with 70% isopropyl alcohol.
- Keeping the swab in place to reduce the risk of cutting your fingers, grasp the ampule on each side of the neck, between the thumb and index finger.
- Quickly snap the ampule at the neck by pushing outward with the thumbs. If there is resistance, rotate the ampule slightly to locate a weaker point. Ampules should not be broken towards the HEPA filter nor towards other sterile products in the hood.
- It is necessary to filter the liquid from an ampule as glass particulates may have fallen into the ampule upon opening. A needle with a 5 micron filter in the hub may be used to filter the liquid either as it is pulled into the syringe or expelled from the syringe but not both ways on the same procedure.
- Tilt the ampule to approximately a 20° degree angle. Surface tension will keep the liquid from spilling out of the ampule.
- Insert the needle into the ampule and place near the opening, bevel facing down; do not touch the opening with the needle.
- To withdraw the ampule contents, pull back the plunger with the thumb of the same hand holding the syringe and without touching the plunger barrel.
- After withdrawing the ampule contents, tap the syringe to move air bubbles to the needle end and expel any excess air.
- Expel any excess fluid back into the ampule.
- If a filter needle were initially used, cap the filter needle, remove and replace with a regular needle when done.
- If a regular needle was initially used, cap the regular needle, remove and replace with a filter needle when done.

Medication Transfer to a Flexible Plastic Intravenous Container

The following steps allow for proper technique for drug additive transfer to a flexible plastic intravenous container utilizing a syringe and needle.

- Only materials necessary for the preparation process should be placed in the hood.
- After withdrawing the necessary amount of drug liquid from a vial or ampule, cap the needle and set the syringe aside.
- Remove the plastic overwrap, which limits fluid loss, from the container.
- The medication, or injection port of the container, should be positioned towards the HEPA filter and swabbed with 70% isopropyl alcohol.
- Uncap the needle, and insert it into the medication port, bevel side facing up, and through the diaphragm. To facilitate this process, the medication port must be fully extended, minimizing puncturing of the side of the port. Also, the needle gauge must be no less than 19 to allow for resealing of the medication port and greater than 3/8 inch in length to allow for complete puncturing of the diaphragm.
- Expel the contents of the syringe.
- Remove syringe and needle and dispose of them properly.
- Gently squeeze or shake the container and inspect.
- Although not necessary, a protective cap or seal may be placed on the medication port to prevent further addition of any medication or tampering.
- Label appropriately.

Medication Transfer to a Glass Intravenous Container

Although flexible plastic intravenous containers are more common, it may be necessary to use a glass intravenous container. This usually occurs when compatibility and stability issues are minimized using glass. The following steps allow for proper technique of drug additive transfer to a glass intravenous container utilizing a syringe and needle.

- Only materials necessary for the preparation process should be placed in the hood.
- After withdrawing the necessary amount of drug liquid from a vial or ampule, cap the needle and set the syringe aside.
- Remove the protective cover from the container by grasping the metal outer tab, pulling down, and then pulling around. Remove the flat metal disc with your fingers to uncover the rubber stopper.
- Swab the rubber stopper with 70% isopropyl alcohol using several firm quick stokes in the same direction.
- Uncap the needle and place the needle tip on the rubber stopper, over the entry port (marking), with the bevel side facing up.
- Insert the needle by straightening the needle out to parallel to the container while pushing through the rubber stopper.
- Expel the contents of the syringe by depressing the plunger or allowing the vacuum to pull in the medication.
- Remove needle and dispose of needle and syringe properly.
- Gently shake the container and inspect.
- Place a protective cap or seal over the rubber stopper to prevent further addition of medication and tampering.
- Label appropriately.

Medication Transfer to a Syringe

Medication may be dispensed in a syringe for direct injection or for use as part of a syringe piggyback system for intravenous infusion. The following steps allow for proper technique when preparing medication for administration from syringes.

- Only materials necessary for the preparation process should be placed in the hood.
- After withdrawing the necessary amount of drug liquid from a vial or ampule, cap the needle and set the syringe aside. The size of syringe used must be appropriate for the type of technique in which the syringe is to be utilized.
- Remove the protective overwrap from a tray of syringe caps.
- Cap and remove needle from syringe and set aside.
- Push syringe tip down onto syringe cap until secure, being careful not to touch syringe tip or cap with your fingers.
- Dispose of needle properly.
- Label appropriately.

Medication Transfer to an Irrigation Bottle

The following steps allow for proper technique for drug additive transfer to an irrigation bottle.

- Only materials necessary for the preparation process should be placed in the hood.
- After withdrawing the necessary amount of drug liquid from a vial or ampule, cap the needle, and set the syringe aside.
- Remove the screw cap from the irrigation bottle, and set aside.
- Uncap the needle, and expel contents of syringe into bottle. Some medications may require filtering to remove particulates and microorganisms. If this occurs, place an appropriate filter on the syringe tip before adding the additive liquid to the irrigating solution.
- Replace screw cap and gently shake solution.
- Dispose of needle and syringe (filter) properly.
- Label appropriately.

LABELING REQUIREMENTS

Once a sterile product has been prepared, it must be properly labeled. It is recommended that the following information appear on each label:

- Patient's name and location.
- Patient's unique identification number.
- Product sequence number for patient or other control number.
- Solution name and volume, or if a syringe is used, indicate the volume of the syringe.
- Additive name(s) and amount(s).
- Date and time of preparation.
- Date and time of expiration.
- Administration date and time.

- Administration directions: frequency, duration, rate.
- Name or initials of person preparing product.
- Name or initials of person checking product.
- Ancillary precautions as labels or typed on label, if applicable.
- Special storage instructions, if applicable.

INSPECTING FINAL STERILE PRODUCT

After completion of the sterile product preparation, a final inspection of the product and supplies should be conducted to verify accuracy of the preparation. It is recommended that the following steps take place to verify an accurately prepared sterile product.

- Check all emptied ampules, vials, bags and bottles for correct size, volume, strength and quantity used.
- Check the final product for clarity, particulate matter and color changes.
- Check the final container for any leaks or cracks.
- Check to ensure that the final product is appropriately labeled.

Compatibility and Stability

The compatibility and stability of drugs in solution is another important aspect of sterile product preparation. Generally, sterile products are prepared in advance of when they are to be administered to the patient. Therefore, it is important to know and check the stability and avoid incompatibilities of the final product. Sterile products should not be prepared until this information is known or has been checked. Such information is routinely available from several sources, including the package insert for the drug additive. One important factor that affects stability is the final concentration of the drug in solution. As a general rule, the more concentrated the final solution, the less stable it is, and the greater the chances of such problems as precipitation and decomposition.

Another important factor affecting compatibility and stability is the pH of the preparation. On the pH scale of 1-14, an acidic product has a pH of less than 7 and an alkaline product has a pH of greater than 7. The farther the number is from 7, the more acidic or alkaline the product. The pH is very important with respect to the problems of precipitation and decomposition.

ANTINEOPLASTIC MEDICATIONS— SPECIAL CONSIDERATIONS

Extra precaution must be used when preparing antineoplastic (chemotherapy) medications. Contact of these products with the skin may result in local tissue damage and extreme irritation to the skin, eyes, nose and mouth. Personnel charged with the responsibility of preparing these products must demonstrate appropriate manipulative technique and use special equipment. The following considerations are intended as additional guidelines for the preparation of antineoplastic medications.

- After appropriate handwashing, put on a disposable gown (closed front, long sleeves, closed cuff) and two pairs of latex gloves.
- Work only in a biological safety cabinet (BSC).
- Disinfect work surface.
- Assemble all material for preparation to reduce leaving and reentering work area.

- Place a disposable, plastic-backed liner on surface of work area to absorb any small spills. This liner should be replaced when significant spillage occurs or at the end of each production sequence.

- Place only items necessary for preparation on the work surface. Remember, the air flow is vertical. Do not place items where they may block the downward flow of air.

- Position yourself so that the front viewing shield of the BSC is at the required access opening and protects your eyes and face.

- Handle all sterile items well inside the BSC, and work at least 3 inches from each side wall.

- Attach and prime I.V. administration sets to I.V. containers prior to adding drug.

- Use only syringes and I.V. administration sets with Leur-lock fittings.

- When removing drug from a vial or an ampule, be sure to use a syringe that is large enough so that the plunger will not separate from the barrel when filled.

- When withdrawing drug solution from a vial, maintain negative pressure inside the vial to prevent solution from leaking out around the needle as it is withdrawn.

- When constituting a vial, insert the needle into the vial top and draw back the plunger to create a slight negative pressure inside the vial by drawing air into the syringe. Slowly inject small amounts of diluent and withdraw equal amounts of air. Keep the needle inside the vial and carefully swirl to dissolve contents, if needed. Invert vial and slowly withdraw solution while exchanging equal volumes of air for solution. Excess solution should remain in the vial. With the vial in an upright position, remove fluid from needle and hub by drawing a small amount of air from the vial and remove needle from vial.

- When removing drug solution from an ampule, draw solution through a 5-micron filter needle and clear solution from the needle and hub. Exchange filter needle for a regular needle, and eject any air and excess solution into an empty sterile vial or non-splash collection vessel.

- If drug solution is transferred to an I.V. bag, wipe injection port, container and administration set with a moist gauze.

- If drug solution is to be dispensed in a syringe, make sure you clear drug solution from hub before removing needle and replacing with a locking cap. Wipe syringe with a moist gauze.

- The I.V. container or syringe is to be placed in a sealable plastic bag prior to dispensing so that any leakage will be contained.

- All used materials are to be placed in plastic sealable bags along with outer pair of gloves. Seal all waste containers inside the BSC.

- Remove and dispose of gown, followed by inner pair of gloves. Do not touch the fingertips of the gloves to skin when removing gloves.

- Wash your hands after glove removal.

The proper use of the laminar airflow hood and the adherence to strict aseptic technique are the two most important factors in the prevention of contamination of sterile products. The exact role of the technician in preparing sterile products will vary according to a state's laws governing the practice of pharmacy and to the practice setting. However, the technician must be a highly motivated, meticulous person who works closely with the pharmacist, who is responsible for supervising and checking the technician's activities. The pharmacy technician is an integral part of the preparation of pharmacy-prepared sterile products.

UNIT III

Calculations for the Pharmacy Tech

Chapter 8
TIPS FOR PROBLEM SOLVING

In this chapter:
- *The Technician and Pharmacy Math*
- *Tips for Problem Solving*
- *How to Cancel Units*

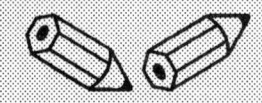

THE TECHNICIAN AND PHARMACY MATH

While many students have grown up comfortable with, or even embracing, technical math, there are probably just as many who have not.

Therefore, the following sections have taken certain artistic license with definitions and equation arrangement in the hope that this presentation will more accurately mesh with the way students naturally think. All alterations of conventional equation arrangement have been designed so that the student will be able to understand and use the information in practice easily and without error.

The pharmacy technician will carry out numerous calculations every day he or she practices. By becoming fluent in the use of pharmaceutical math, the technician will be able to practice safely and easily.

In some of the chapters, shortcuts will be provided after an explanation of a more mathematically correct version. These shortcuts are provided for two reasons:

- An understanding of the correct process may short-circuit the numerous incorrect, and sometimes not so short, shortcuts that are shown to new technicians by co-workers.
- I am hopeful that, by showing the shortcut after the more lengthy version, the technician will more fully understand the reason for performing the calculation and that this knowledge will boost the technician's confidence in his or her other calculations as well.

TIPS FOR SUCCESSFUL PROBLEM-SOLVING

Multiple methods can be employed to accomplish most tasks. Not all of these methods are correct, however, and among those which are, some are correct but very time-consuming, while others are both correct and expedient. The student of technical math must choose among various correct, easy ways of solving problems. By learning the principles behind the formulas, each individual can find the method of solving problems which works best for him or her. Specifically, the student should attempt to answer the questions, "What are we trying to find?" and "Why are we trying to find it?" Armed with the answers to these two questions and an open mind, the student can find new ways of solving old problems.

This text is only the beginning—a means of collecting the very basics of experience. One should continually look for new and faster ways of solving problems without sacrificing accuracy.

Points to Remember

- The very first step in problem solving is data collection. In this phase, determine **what you have** and **what you want**. Since this phase will often include a lot of unnecessary data, one should then separate out **what you need**.

- By conducting these steps first, mental clutter can be minimized and the chances for obtaining an accurate solution are increased.

- **What you need** will have units attached to it. By studying the units needed for the final answer, the student will find it easier to arrange any equation so that these are the only units that appear after all cancelling has been done.

How to Cancel Units

An oversimplified but easy way to remember how units cancel can be stated as follows:

"Any unit, divided by itself, becomes 1 or disappears."

Example:

$$\frac{1}{4 \text{ Liter}} \times 1 \text{ Liter} = \frac{1 \text{ Liter}}{4 \text{ liter}} \text{ or } 1 \text{ Liter} \div 4 \text{ Liter} \rightarrow \frac{1}{4}$$

Answer: $\frac{1}{4}$

As illustrated by the above example, one may multiply two numbers to achieve unit cancellation if one or both of these numbers are expressed as a fraction.

Another way to create cancellation is to consider converting what you have to other similar units which appear in the final answer (i.e. converting minutes to hours or meters to centimeters).

Example:

Convert 120 minutes to hours:

Solution:

$$120 \text{ minutes} \times \frac{1 \text{ hour}}{60 \text{ minutes}} = \frac{120 \text{ hour}}{60} \text{ or } 2 \text{ hours}$$

Even though we more commonly say "There are 60 minutes in 1 hour," we may also say "There is 1 hour in 60 minutes." Both expressions are correct; they are merely different ways of expressing quantities.

A Note About the Value of Mental Calculations

In this age of electronic calculators, some of us have become unaccustomed to doing mental math because we do not feel that it is necessary. While mental calculations **are** unnecessary to obtain a correct answer quickly and accurately, doing mental math yields benefits that extend beyond obtaining the correct answer. By honing the skills necessary to solve problems mentally rather than electronically, many individuals will develop a better ability to find **what you have** and **what you want** from data that is collected.

Certainly, mental calculations do not have to be done for every problem, but they should be attempted consistently for maximum benefit.

With this said, let us begin our adventure!

Chapter 9
THE LANGUAGE OF PHARMACY

In this chapter:
- *Learning the Language*
- *Roman Numerals*
- *Latin Abbreviations and their Meanings*

LEARNING THE LANGUAGE

As each nation has its own language, so does each profession. The language of health care is a hodge-podge of archaic numbering and measuring systems, dead languages and abbreviations. As we move towards the 21st Century, reason is beginning to prevail and one true standard is developing. However, there are still those who insist on doing things in the way to which they have become accustomed. In this and other chapters, you will be presented with the most commonly used facets of the traditional system

Roman Numerals

Although the more familiar Arabic system is most commonly used, many health care professionals still use the Roman system occasionally. There are only eight numerals in this system:

- ss
- L
- I
- C
- V
- D
- X
- M

Their values are defined in the table on page 74.

Roman Numerals and Arabic Equivalents

ROMAN NUMERAL	ARABIC EQUIVALENT
ss	½
I	1
V	5
X	10
L	50
C	100
D	500
M	1,000

Points to Remember

Numbers other than these eight are created according to the following rules:

- With the exception of M, no numeral may be repeated more than three times in a row.
  - **Example:** III is correct, but IIII is not.
- When a smaller numeral is on the right of a larger or equal numeral, the numerals are added.
  - **Example:** VI = 6, XI = 11, XV = 15, XX = 20
- When a larger numeral is to the right of a small numeral, the smaller numeral is subtracted from the larger.
  - **Example:** IX = 9, XL = 40, IV = 4, CD = 400
- Rules 2 and 3 may be applied together to form any number.
  - **Example:** MCXL = 1,140

In this example, the first two numerals (MC = 1,000 + 100 = 1,100) followed Rule 2 and the second two numerals (XL = 50 − 10 = 40) followed Rule 3. The product of the second two numerals was smaller than the first two numerals, so it was added.

Abbreviations

In addition to the use of Roman numerals, traditional pharmaceutical language utilizes instructions in the form of abbreviated Latin words and phrases.

The most commonly used abbreviations are listed in the table on page 75. To limit rampant use of non-traditional abbreviations, institutions such as hospitals sometimes restrict the use of abbreviations to a manageable list. The most important abbreviations to know are those dealing with frequency (i.e. b.i.d) and route (i.e. p.o.).

Latin Abbreviations and Their Meanings

LATIN ABBREVIATION	MEANING
a.c	before meals
ad	up to (do not confuse with a.d.!)
a.d.	right ear
ad lib.	as desired
amp	ampule
a.s.	left ear
a.u.	both ears
b.i.d.	twice daily
BSA	body surface area
$\bar{c}$	with
cap	capsule
cc	cubic centimeter
$\overline{cc}$	with meals
dc or d/c	discontinue
D$_5$W	5% dextrose in water
fl	fluid
g or gm	gram
gr	grain
gtt	drop
inj	injection
I.V	intravenous
IVPB or PB	intravenous piggyback
m^2	square meter
I.M	intramuscular
h.s.	at bedtime
mcg	microgram
mEq	milliequivalent
mg	milligram
ml	milliliter
n/v	nausea and/or vomiting
n.p.o	nothing by mouth

NS	normal saline
o.d.	right eye
o.s.	left eye
o.u.	both eyes
p.c.	after meals
p.o.	by mouth
prn	as necessary or as needed
q.d.	each day
q.i.d.	four times daily
q.o.d.	every other day
q.s.	a sufficient quantity
pr	by rectum
s̄	without
sc or sq	subcutaneously
susp	suspension
tab	tablet
tbsp	tablespoon
t.i.d.	three times daily
tsp	teaspoon
u	unit
u.d. or ut dict	as directed
ung.	ointment

Often these abbreviations are modified by the individual writing them; the modifications come primarily in the form of deletion of periods. This personalization of abbreviations should be kept in mind when interpreting any drug order.

❖ PRACTICE PROBLEMS

1. List the eight Roman numerals.

2. List the Arabic equivalent of the following Roman numerals:
    a. XV   **b.** ssV   **c.** IX   **d.** XXXV (or VXL)
    e. MCVL   **f.** CVL   **g.** XIV   **h.** VD
    i. XVss

3. Give the Latin abbreviation for the following:
    a. nothing by mouth
    b. before meals
    c. by rectum
    d. teaspoonful
    e. both ears
    f. four times daily
    g. three times daily
    h. two times daily
    i. once daily
    j. left eye
    k. right eye
    l. by mouth

4. Convert the following Arabic numerals to Roman numerals:
    a. 23   **b.** 16   **c.** 55   **d.** 99
    e. 106   **f.** 501   **g.** 550   **h.** 900
    i. 1100   **j.** 2000   **k.** 3500

5. Convert the following Roman numerals to their Arabic equivalents:
    a. XXI   **b.** XL   **c.** LXVI   **d.** XC
    e. CLXVI   **f.** CCL   **g.** MX   **h.** MLX
    i. DXL   **j.** XD   **k.** MMX

Chapter 10
FRACTIONS

In this chapter:
- *Enlarging and Reducing Fractions*
- *Addition and Subtraction of Fractions*
- *Multiplying and Dividing Fractions*
- *Calculators and Fractions*

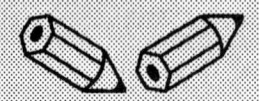

DEFINING FRACTIONS

The pharmaceuticals currently being used by health care professionals are so potent that doses are often measured in fractions of a whole number. Therefore, it is important for the technician to be able to manipulate fractions easily.

All fractions have two components: a numerator and a denominator. In the case of decimal fractions, the numerator and denominator are expressed differently and will be discussed later. The structure of fractions is as follows:

$$\frac{\text{numerator}}{\text{denominator}}$$

Points to Remember

There are two types of fractions: common and decimal.

- Common fractions may be further broken down into the following:

    - Proper — in which the numerator is less than the denominator, i.e. $\frac{1}{2}$

    - Improper — where the numerator is greater than the denominator: $\frac{8}{7}$

    - Mixed — a combination of a whole number and a fraction: $1\frac{2}{3}$

    - Complex — the numerator and the denominator are both fractions: $\frac{1/7}{1/6}$

- Decimal fractions are numbers in which the denominator is expressed as a decimal point instead of as a number. Each space to the left reflects an increase in the denominator by a power of 10.

Examples

$$0.1 = \frac{1}{10}, \quad 0.01 = \frac{1}{100}, \quad 0.001 = \frac{1}{1000}$$

A decimal is simply the number that results from dividing the numerator by the denominator.

$$\frac{1}{10} \rightarrow 1 \div 10 = 0.1, \quad \frac{2}{10} \rightarrow 2 \div 10 = 0.2$$

An important point to remember: Always place the zero in front of the decimal point. This should be done to avoid confusion over the placement or even the existence of the decimal point, i.e., 0.5 could be interpreted as 5 or 0.5 depending on how well the decimal was made. It is easy to see the harm that could be caused!

ENLARGING AND REDUCING FRACTIONS

There are many occasions in which a fraction in a given problem will need to be altered to make the solution to that problem easier. Fractions may be enlarged or reduced "as long as the numerator and the denominator are altered by the same multiplier or divisor." By manipulating both the numerator and the denominator in this manner, the numeric value of the fraction is unchanged. The key is to duplicate what you have done to both numerator and denominator.

The only allowable arithmetic functions are division and multiplication, as addition or subtraction would change the value of the fraction.

Enlarging Fractions

Enlarging is often necessary when adding or subtracting fractions. Both the numerator and denominator are multiplied by a number of you or your instructor's choosing. Fractions are enlarged to create a "common denominator." (Common denominators will be discussed in the next section.)

✍ CHECK YOUR UNDERSTANDING

1. Convert $\frac{2}{3}$ to $\frac{x}{6}$

a. Since 6 is 2 times larger than 3, the denominator (3) must be multiplied by 2.

b. Since the denominator has been multiplied by 2, the numerator must also be multiplied by 2. $\quad \frac{2 \times 2}{3 \times 2} = \frac{4}{6}$

Answer: $\frac{4}{6}$

80 Fractions

2. Convert $\frac{1}{9}$ to $\frac{3}{x}$

a.   To change the numerator to 3, the original numerator must be multiplied by 3.

b.   Since the numerator was multiplied by 3, so must the denominator. $\frac{1 \times 3}{9 \times 3} = \frac{3}{27}$

Answer: $\frac{3}{27}$

Reducing Fractions

Fractions will normally be reduced after the final solution has been achieved. Normally the answer will be requested to be placed in "lowest terms." This means that the fraction has been reduced as much as possible.

To reduce to lower terms, one must find the **largest** number by which both numerator and denominator can be divided. Both the numerator and denominator are then divided by that number.

✍ CHECK YOUR UNDERSTANDING

1. Reduce 3/27 to lowest terms:

a.   Both numerator and denominator can be divided by 3.

b: $\frac{3}{27} \div \frac{3}{3} = \frac{1}{9}$

Answer: $\frac{1}{9}$

2. Reduce 2/6 to lowest terms:

a.   Both numerator and denominator are divisible by 2.

b. $\frac{2}{6} \div \frac{2}{2} = \frac{1}{3}$

Answer: $\frac{1}{3}$

If the numerator of the answer is greater than the denominator, then the answer is greater than 1. If this occurs, you may be asked to do one of two things:

   1. Leave the number as an improper fraction
   2. Reduce to a mixed fraction.

When asked to express the answer as a mixed fraction, divide the numerator by the denominator, write down the whole number produced and leave the remainder expressed as a fraction.

3. Reduce 26/4 to a mixed fraction.

a.   Divide 26 by 4

b.   26 ÷ 4 = 6, remainder 2

Answer: $6\frac{2}{4}$ or $6\frac{1}{2}$

ADDING AND SUBTRACTING FRACTIONS

Addition and subtraction of fractions requires that all fractions involved have a "common denominator." That is, all denominators in the equation must be the same number. The fractions 1/3 and 2/3 have a common denominator and may be added or subtracted without further alteration. However, 1/3 and 2/7 do not share a common denominator and thus must be enlarged. The quickest way to convert 1/3 and 2/7 to fractions having a common denominator is to multiply the denominators by each other.

$$3 \times 7 = 21$$

Next the numerators must be enlarged appropriately:

$$\frac{1 \times 7}{3 \times 7} = \frac{7}{21}$$

$$\frac{2 \times 3}{7 \times 3} = \frac{6}{21}$$

The final fractions will look like this:

$$\frac{7}{21} + \frac{6}{21}$$

The reader is asked to consult the section on Enlarging and Reducing Fractions on page 79 if this in unclear.

After conversion to a common denominator, the numerators are then added or subtracted, depending on the equation. The denominator does not change until this operation is carried out. After the answer is found, it may be reduced to lowest terms, if appropriate.

✎ CHECK YOUR UNDERSTANDING

1. Find the sum of $\frac{1}{3} + \frac{8}{13}$

   a. Find a common denominator—$3 \times 13 = 39$

   b. Enlarge both fractions based on the new denominator:

   $$\frac{1 \times 13}{3 \times 13} = \frac{13}{39} \qquad \frac{8 \times 3}{13 \times 3} = \frac{24}{39}$$

   c. Solve based on new fractions:

   $$\frac{13}{39} + \frac{24}{39} = \frac{37}{39}$$

   d. **Reduce:** No reduction is possible.

2. Find the sum of $\frac{1}{2} + \frac{1}{16}$

   a. Find the common denominator—$2 \times 16 = 32$

   b. Enlarge both fractions:

   $$\frac{1 \times 16}{2 \times 16} = \frac{16}{32} \qquad \frac{1 \times 2}{16 \times 2} = \frac{2}{32}$$

   c. **Solve:**

   $$\frac{16}{32} + \frac{2}{32} = \frac{18}{32}$$

d. Reduce: In this case, both numerator and denominator may be divided by 2:

Answer: $\dfrac{18 \div 2}{32 \div 2} = \dfrac{9}{16}$

MULTIPLYING FRACTIONS

No common denominator is needed to multiply fractions; numerators are multiplied by numerators, and denominators are multiplied by denominators.

Example # 1

$$\frac{1}{16} \times \frac{1}{2} \rightarrow \frac{1 \times 1}{16 \times 2} = \frac{1}{32}$$

Example # 2

$$\frac{1}{3} \times \frac{2}{7} \times \frac{3}{8} \rightarrow \frac{1 \times 2 \times 3}{3 \times 7 \times 8} = \frac{6}{168}$$

This can be further reduced by dividing by 6:

$$\frac{6}{168} \div \frac{6}{6} = \frac{1}{28}$$

Answer: $\dfrac{1}{28}$

DIVIDING FRACTIONS

Dividing by a fraction is the **same** as multiplying by the **reciprocal** of that fraction. The following is an example:

$$1 \div \frac{1}{3} \rightarrow 1 \times \frac{3}{1} = 3$$

Further investigation of the problem yields the question: "How many ⅓'s are in 1." The solution is how many ⅓ portions can be created from 1 whole number. Since ⅜ = 1, the answer is 3.

✍ CHECK YOUR UNDERSTANDING

1. Find the quotient: $2 \div \dfrac{2}{3}$

a. How many $\dfrac{2}{3}$ portions are in 2?

b. $2 \times \dfrac{3}{2} = \dfrac{6}{2}$

c Reduce $\dfrac{6}{2} \rightarrow 3$

Answer: 3

2. Find the quotient: $3 \div \frac{1}{2}$

a. How many $\frac{1}{2}$ portions can be created from 3?

b. $3 \times \frac{2}{1} = \frac{6}{1}$ **or** 6

Answer: 6

CALCULATORS AND FRACTIONS

The age of technology has brought many important advancements—one of the most important being the hand-held calculator. This little piece of microcircuitry has changed the way we do math and the way we express fractions.

Calculators will display and calculate fractions only as some multiple of ten expressed as a decimal. Thus, $\frac{1}{6}$ becomes 0.1666 or 0.167.

To convert a decimal from the calculator display into a fraction on paper:

1. Place the number found on the display in the numerator **without** the decimal point.
2. Count the numbers found behind the decimal point on the display. Attach this same quantity of zeros to the numeral 1 to create the denominator.

✍ CHECK YOUR UNDERSTANDING

1. Convert 0.2 to a workable fraction

a. Place a 2 where the numerator belongs.

b. Place a 1 with 1 zero (10) where the denominator belongs.

Answer: $\frac{2}{10}$ **reduce** $\frac{1}{5}$

2. Convert 0.125 to a workable fraction.

a. Numerator = 125

b. Denominator = 1000 (three decimal points in 0.125)

Answer: $\frac{125}{1000}$ **reduce** $\frac{1}{8}$

3. Convert 0.25 to a workable fraction.

a. Numerator = 25

b. Denominator = 100 (two decimal places in 0.25)

Answer: $\frac{25}{100}$ **reduce** $\frac{1}{4}$

To convert a fraction to a decimal: Divide the numerator by the denominator.

4. *Convert ¼ to a decimal*
   1 ÷ 4 = 0.25

❖ PRACTICE PROBLEMS

1. *Which of the following is a proper fraction?*
   a. $\frac{3}{2}$ b. $1\frac{1}{7}$ c. $\frac{1}{6}$ d. $\frac{6}{3}$

2. Of the numbers above, which is a mixed fraction?

3. Express 0.3 as a proper fraction.

4. Enlarge $\frac{1}{3}$ to a fraction having the form $\frac{x}{9}$.

5. Reduce $\frac{3}{39}$ to lowest terms.

6. *Solve the following:*
   a. $\frac{1}{3} + \frac{1}{6}$ b. $\frac{13}{16} - \frac{3}{8}$ c. $\frac{2}{3} \times \frac{3}{7}$ d. $\frac{7}{8} \div \frac{1}{3}$

7. Enlarge $\frac{6}{7}$ to $\frac{x}{49}$

8. Reduce $\frac{4}{16}$ to $\frac{x}{4}$

9. *Solve:*
   a. $\frac{1}{16} + \frac{4}{16}$ b. $\frac{1}{8} \times \frac{5}{7}$ c. $\frac{8}{9} \div \frac{1}{2}$ d. $1\frac{1}{8} - \frac{5}{16}$

10. Convert $2\frac{1}{3}$ to an improper fraction.

11. Convert $\frac{16}{5}$ to a mixed fraction.

12. Convert 0.125 to a proper fraction.

13. Convert 0.45 to proper fraction.

14. Convert $\frac{59}{17}$ to a mixed fraction.

15. *Add the following:*
    a. $\frac{1}{2} + \frac{1}{3}$ b. $\frac{3}{16} + \frac{9}{7}$

16. *Subtract the following:*
    a. $\frac{97}{100} - \frac{1}{6} - \frac{2}{5}$ b. $\frac{13}{16} - \frac{1}{5} - \frac{1}{4}$

17. *Multiply the following:*
    a. $\frac{8}{9} \times \frac{1}{3}$ b. $\frac{11}{21} \times \frac{2}{5}$

18. *Divide the following:*
    a. $\frac{9}{16} \div \frac{1}{2}$ b. $\frac{3}{5} \div \frac{1}{5}$

Chapter 11
THE METRIC SYSTEM

In this chapter:
- *Units of Metric Measurement*
- *Metric Abbreviations*
- *Conversions of Metric Measurement*

UNITS OF METRIC MEASUREMENT

Almost all measurements of weight, volume and length in health care are conducted utilizing the metric system. This system of weights and measures has risen to prominence due to its simplicity.

Points to Remember

- All measurements of weight, volume and length are named according to the same basic rules, and each measurement has a prefix which denotes the magnitude of a quantity relative to a base term.
- The suffix denotes whether the measurement is of weight, volume or length.
- The suffix is also the base term.

Metric Terms and What They Measure

Metric Base Term	Abbreviation	What It Measures
gram	g	weight
liter	l	volume
meter	m	length

Metric Length

The base unit of metric length is the meter. The word *meter* appears as a suffix in all words designating measurements greater or less than one meter.

Metric Volume

The base term of volume is the liter, theoretically intended to be 1,000 cubic centimeters (presumably to connect all metric measurements to a common theme).

While modern science has determined that this is not exactly correct, it is so close that the *United States Pharmacopeia* has determined that cubic centimeter and milliliter may be used interchangeably.

Metric Weight

The base unit of weight is the gram, the weight of one cubic centimeter of water at 4° centigrade.

Metric Abbreviations

Abbreviated units of metric measurement are composed the same way as in long form, that is, the abbreviated prefix is added to the abbreviation of the base term.

Metric Prefixes and Relative Values

METRIC PREFIX	ABBREVIATION	VALUE RELATIVE TO THE BASE TERM
myria		10,000 times
kilo	k	1,000 times
hekto	h	100 times
deka	da	10 times
Base Term		**1 time**
deci	d	one tenth
centi	c	one hundredth
milli	m	one thousandth
micro	mc	one millionth
nano	n	one billionth
pico	p	one trillionth

CHECK YOUR UNDERSTANDING

Refer to the *Metric Prefixes and Relative Values* chart on the preceding page to answer the following questions.

1. Find the correct nomenclature for ¹⁄1000 of a meter:

a. ¹⁄1000 meter = milli

b. base term = meter

c. milli + meter = millimeter

2. Name ¹⁄100 of a meter appropriately:

a. ¹⁄100 = centi

b. base term = meter

c. centi + meter = centimeter

3. Name one billionth of a meter according to the rules laid out previously:

a. 1 billionth of base term = nano

b. base term = meter

c. nano + meter = nanometer

CONVERSIONS OF METRIC MEASUREMENT

Often, a metric quantity will need to be reduced or enlarged to make that quantity easier to calculate or to make an answer take a practical form.

CHECK YOUR UNDERSTANDING

1. Convert 20,000 mg to grams:

Using Dimensional Analysis

$$20,000 \text{ mg} \times \frac{1 \text{ gram}}{1,000 \text{ mg}} = \frac{20,000 \text{ grams}}{1000} \rightarrow 20 \text{ grams}$$

Answer: 20 grams

Using Proportion

$$\frac{20,000 \text{ mg}}{x \text{ g}} = \frac{1000 \text{ mg}}{1 \text{ gram}}$$

$$1,000x = 20,000$$

Answer: x = 20 grams

2. Convert 0.1 liter to ml:

Dimensional Analysis

$$0.1 \text{ L} \times \frac{1000 \text{ ml}}{\text{L}} = 100 \text{ ml}$$

Answer: 100 ml

Proportion

$$\frac{0.1 \text{ L}}{x \text{ ml}} = \frac{1 \text{ L}}{1,000 \text{ ml}}$$

Answer: x = 100 ml

❖ PRACTICE PROBLEMS

Give the correct name for the following:

1. 1,000 grams
2. One-millionth of a liter
3. 10 meters
4. One-trillionth of a gram

What are the proper abbreviations for the following:

5. Picogram
6. Milliliter
7. Kilometer
8. Deciliter
9. Nanogram
10. Centimeter

Convert:

11. 1500 meters to kilometers
12. 40,000 milliliters to liters
13. 8,000 grams to kilograms
14. One billion picograms to grams
15. 125 micrograms to milligrams

Chapter 12
APOTHECARIES' AND AVOIRDUPOIS SYSTEMS OF MEASUREMENT

In this chapter:
- *Apothecaries' System of Measurement*
- *Avoirdupois System of Measurement*
- *Conversion of Units of Differing Systems*

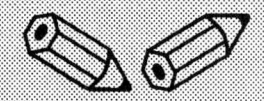

UNDERSTANDING THE SYSTEMS

The Apothecaries' and Avoirdupois systems have largely fallen out of use in the medical community, although certain units are still used in commerce. To prevent errors due to misinterpretation, the student should, at least, be able to identify units of both systems. It is also most helpful to know that items in commerce, i.e., bulk chemicals bought from a warehouse, will be measured by Avoirdupois units, whereas compounding in the pharmacy will be conducted according to Apothecaries' units!

To simplify this process, measurements in Apothecaries' units will be followed by this designator: (apoth). Additionally, Avoirdupois measurements will be followed by: (avoir). Later sections will deal with the conversion of these units among themselves and to the metric system.

Apothecaries' System of Fluid Measurement

- 60 minims = 1 fluidram
- 16 fluidounces = 1 pint (pt)
- 4 quarts = 1 gallon (gal)
- 8 fluidrams = 1 fluidounce
- 2 pints = 1 quart (qt)

As may be apparent, the units *ounce, pint, quart,* and *gallon* are still commonly used in the United States.

Apothecaries' System of Weight

- 20 grains (gr) = 1 scruple
- 8 drams = 1 ounce
- 3 scruples = 1 dram
- 12 ounces = 1 pound (lb)

NOTE: The units dram and ounce appear in **both** the weight and volume systems with the only difference being the addition of the designator "fluid" or "f" for liquid measurement. When it is readily apparent that a liquid is to be measured, many physicians and pharmacists will drop the "fluid" designator. If there is any confusion as to whether a solid or fluid is to be measured, the units must be clarified as the fluidram and the dram are quite different.

Avoirdupois System of Weight Measurement

- 437.5 grains (gr) = 1 ounce
- 16 ounces (oz) = 1 pound (lb)

NOTE: Both Apothecaries' and Avoirdupois systems use the grain, ounce, and pound. However, only the grain has the same weight in both systems. This latter fact becomes useful when converting between systems.

ERROR PREVENTION ALERT:
The abbreviation for grain (gr) is sometimes used incorrectly to denote grams (g); awareness of this fact may be used to prevent many potentially serious errors. A clue to the correct use of the grain abbreviation lies with the placement of the abbreviation in relation to the quantity. When the grain abbreviation is used correctly, it will be placed in front of the numeral which denotes the quantity of substance being measured.

Example

a. gr X is correct and denotes a 10 grain quantity
b. 10 gr is incorrect, but more than likely means 10 grains. This example would need clarification, as it could also mean 10 grams.
c. gr 10 is correct also (although gr X is more common).

Common Metric, Apothecaries' and Avoirdupois Equivalents

METRIC	APOTHECARIES'
1 milliliter	16.23 minims (apoth)
3.69 ml	1 fluidram (apoth)
29.57 (or 30) ml	1 fluidounce (apoth)
473 ml	1 pint (apoth)
3785 ml	1 gallon (apoth)
1 kilogram	2.2 pounds (avoir)
454 grams	1 pound (avoir)

373.2 grams	1 pound (apoth)
1 oz. (avoir)	437.5 gr
65 or 60 mg	1 grain
1 gram	15.432 grains

NOTE: There are two correct equivalents for the quantity of milligrams per grain. The conversion is inconsistently applied so experience will dictate as to which conversion is being used.

The Household System

The household system contains only two significant units: the teaspoon and the tablespoon. The metric equivalents of these units are listed below.

Unit	Household Measure Equivalent
teaspoon	5 ml
tablespoon	15 ml

CONVERSION OF UNITS OF DIFFERING SYSTEMS

1. Convert the given quantity to grains
2. Reduce this grain quantity to units of the desired system. (This may require multiple steps.)

✍ CHECK YOUR UNDERSTANDING

1. Convert 2 oz (avoir) to Apothecaries' measure:

1. $2 \text{ oz} \times \dfrac{435 \text{ grains}}{\text{ounce (avoir)}} = 875 \text{ grains}$

2. a. $875 \text{ grains} \times \dfrac{1 \text{ scruple}}{20 \text{ grains}} \times \dfrac{1 \text{ dram}}{3 \text{ scruples}} \times \dfrac{1 \text{ ounce}}{8 \text{ drams}} = 1 \text{ oz. (apoth)}$ 395 grain remainder

   b. $395 \text{ grains} \times \dfrac{1 \text{ scruple}}{20 \text{ grains}} \times \dfrac{1 \text{ dram}}{3 \text{ scruples}} = 6 \text{ drams, 35 grain remainder}$

   c. $35 \text{ grains} \times \dfrac{1 \text{ scruple}}{20 \text{ grains}} = 1 \text{ scruple, 15 grain remainder}$

Answer: 1 oz, 6 drams, 1 scruple, 15 grains

As the preceding example shows, an analysis of the grain remainder after each conversion is completed is required. Most often, the only units of concern are pounds, ounces and grains. If this were true for the example, one could have stopped after the initial operation and given 1 ounce, 395 grains as the answer.

2. Convert 1 pound (avoir) to Apothecaries' measure:

1. $1 \text{ pound} \times \dfrac{16 \text{ ounces}}{1 \text{ pound}} \times \dfrac{437.5 \text{ grains}}{\text{ounce}} = 7000 \text{ grains}$

92 Apothecaries' and Avoirdupois Systems

2. a. $7000 \text{ grains} \times \dfrac{\text{scruple}}{20 \text{ grains}} \times \dfrac{\text{dram}}{3 \text{ scruples}} \times \dfrac{\text{ounce}}{8 \text{ drams}} \times \dfrac{\text{pound}}{12 \text{ ounces}} =$

    1 pound, 1240 grain remainder

    b. $1240 \text{ grains} \times \dfrac{\text{scruple}}{20 \text{ grains}} \times \dfrac{\text{dram}}{3 \text{ scruples}} \times \dfrac{\text{ounce}}{8 \text{ drams}} = 2$ ounces, 280 grain remainder

    c. $280 \text{ grains} \times \dfrac{\text{scruple}}{20 \text{ grains}} \times \dfrac{\text{dram}}{3 \text{ scruples}} = 4$ drams, 40 grain remainder

    d. $40 \text{ grain} \times \dfrac{\text{scruple}}{20 \text{ grains}} = 2$ scruples

Answer: 1 pound, 2 ounces, 4 drams, 2 scruples

An alternative to this lengthy answer is to express to grain remainder after determining pounds as a pound fraction. To illustrate:

1 pound, 1240 grain remainder becomes → 1 pound, $\dfrac{1240 \text{ grains}}{5760 \text{ grains}}$ (apoth)

reduce

$1\dfrac{31}{144}$ pounds (apoth)

or

1.2152 pounds (apoth)

Conversions of Household Units

Since there are only two household units to learn, their conversions are relatively easy. These conversions will be used on a daily basis, so they **must be memorized.**

The conversion factors to **memorize** are:

- 1 teaspoonful (tsp) = 5 ml
- 1 tablespoonful (tbsp) = 15 ml

The following examples will illustrate two methods of arriving at the desired answer:

✍ CHECK YOUR UNDERSTANDING

1. A dose of 2 tbsp is needed. How many ml is this?

Method # 1

$\dfrac{15 \text{ ml}}{\text{Tbsp}} = \dfrac{x \text{ ml}}{2 \text{ Tbsp}}$

x = 30

Answer: 30 ml

Method # 2

$2 \text{ Tbsp} \times \dfrac{15 \text{ ml}}{\text{Tbsp}} = 30 \text{ ml}$

2. A child is to take 3 tsp of a medicine. How many ml is this?

Method # 1

$\dfrac{5 \text{ ml}}{\text{tsp}} = \dfrac{x \text{ ml}}{3 \text{ tsp}}$

x = 15

Answer: 15 ml

Method # 2

$3 \text{ tsp} \times \dfrac{5 \text{ ml}}{\text{tsp}} = 15 \text{ ml}$

❖ PRACTICE PROBLEMS

Convert:

1. 4 pounds (apoth) to Avoirdupois (round to 2 decimal places)
2. 7 pounds (avoir) to Apothecaries'
3. 1 ounce (avoir) to milligrams (two different answers are correct)
4. 5 teaspoonsful to milliliters
5. 2 pints to milliliters
6. 3 gallons to ounces (two different answers are correct)
7. 1 ounce (avoir) to milligrams (two answers are possible)
8. Convert gr X to milligrams (Either conversion is acceptable)
9. One fluid ounce to teaspoonsful
10. 10 ml to teaspoonsful
11. 130 mg to grains
12. 6 teaspoonsful to tablespoonsful
13. gr V to milligrams
14. 14,000 grains to pounds (avoir)
15. 14,000 grains to pounds (apoth)
16. A patient is to take one teaspoonful of medicine three times daily for ten days. How many milliliters are to be dispensed?
17. A patient is to receive gr V of a drug four times daily for 5 days. How many mg of the drug should be dispensed?

94 *Ratio and Proportion*

Chapter 13
RATIO AND PROPORTION

In this chapter:
- *Methods of Calculation*
- *Ratio*
- *Proportion*

METHODS OF CALCULATION

Many of the problems encountered in this text and on the job may be solved by more than one method of calculation. Some methods decrease the time need to find the solution and increase accuracy for certain types of problems, while other methods are better suited for different circumstances.

Points to Remember

- All but the simplest problems may be solved by proportion. This method will be discussed in a later section.
- Another method is a bit more intuitive and has greater utility for experienced calculators. Multiplication or division is carried out on an object numeral by a conversion factor found by surveying the problem.

Examples

1. One kilogram is equal to 2.2 pounds. How many pounds are in 5 kilograms?

a. Since the object numeral is 5 kilograms, our conversion factor must be in pounds. Thus, the conversion factor must be in pounds.

b. The object numeral is multiplied by our conversion factor in this instance because it takes more than 1 pound to make one kilogram.

Answer: 5 × 2.2 = 11 pounds

The units for the answer are pounds because the conversion factor was pounds.

2. 1 pound is equal to 0.454 kilograms. How many kilograms are in 2.2 pounds? (Round to one decimal place.)

a. Our conversion factor becomes 0.454 because our answer is needed in kilograms.

b. The object numeral (2.2) is multiplied by 0.454 in this case because it takes less than 1 kilogram to make a pound.

Answer: 2.2 × 0.454 = 1 kilogram

An easier way of conducting this sort of conversion is accomplished by arranging all the variables in such a way that they cancel each other out when they are multiplied by each other. The following problem provides an example of this method of calculation.

3. One kilogram equals 2.2 pounds. How many pounds are in 5 kilograms?

a. 5 kilograms × $\dfrac{2.2 \text{ pounds}}{1 \text{ kilogram}}$

b. $\dfrac{(5 \text{ kilograms})(2.2 \text{ pounds})}{1 \text{ kilogram}}$

c. Since kilograms are present on the top and bottom of the equation, those units cancel:

$$\dfrac{(5)(2.2 \text{ pounds})}{1}$$

Answer: 5 × 2.2 pounds = 11 pounds

There are fewer rules to remember with this method: The number to be converted begins the equation, and all units except those asked for by the question must cancel.

✍ CHECK YOUR UNDERSTANDING

1. One pound = 0.4545 kilograms. How many kilograms are in 2.2 pounds?

a. 2.2 pounds × $\dfrac{0.4545 \text{ kilograms}}{1 \text{ pound}}$

b. Pounds will cancel:

$$\dfrac{(2.2)(0.4545 \text{ kilograms})}{1} = 0.9999 \text{ kilogram } \textbf{or } 1 \text{ kilogram}$$

2. There are 100 pennies in 1 dollar. How many pennies are in 10 dollars?

a. 10 dollars × $\dfrac{100 \text{ pennies}}{\text{dollar}}$

b. 10 × 100 pennies = 1,000 pennies

Comparison of Methods

Each of the three methods described previously has advantages and disadvantages.

One method may be easier and/or faster than the others when used for a given type of problem, but harder/slower for others. It is most important to choose a method which will allow complete confidence in the answer obtained.

96 *Ratio and Proportion*

✍ CHECK YOUR UNDERSTANDING

There are 100 pennies in one dollar. How many pennies are in 50 dollars? (All three methods will be used to solve the problem.)

Conversion/Proportion

$$\frac{100 \text{ pennies}}{\text{dollar}} = \frac{x \text{ pennies}}{50 \text{ dollars}}$$

$$x = 5000 \text{ pennies}$$

Simplified Conversion/Dimensional Analysis

$$50 \text{ dollars} \times \frac{100 \text{ pennies}}{1 \text{ dollar}} = 5000 \text{ pennies}$$

As should be evident, simple problems are solved more slowly by the proportion method. When problems become more difficult and units harder to track, proportion and dimensional analysis have greater utility in preventing errors.

RATIO AND PROPORTION

In order to utilize the proportion method of calculation, a working knowledge of ratios is necessary. A ratio is the relationship of one quantity to another. It may have the basic appearance of a fraction, or the numerals comprising the ratio may be separated by a colon. Thus, the ratio of a mixture that contains 2 milligrams of atropine for each 1 milligram of scopolamine would be expressed verbally as "2 to 1 ratio" or written 2:1 or ²⁄₁.

Points to Remember

- When the ratio is written as a fraction, it should not be reduced. The reason for this is that a ratio is not a true fraction but an expression of relative quantity.

- Ratios have no units; therefore, the quantities they represent are flexible. Consider the preceding atropine: scopolamine ratio of 2:1; the units attached to this ratio may be changed to suit the needs of the pharmacist or technician.

- If a given quantity of this mixture contains 2 kilograms of atropine, then it also contains 1 kilogram of scopolamine, 2 tons of atropine; the mixture would yield 1 ton of scopolamine, and 2 milligrams of atropine: 1 milligram of scopolamine. If no units are given then this mixture would be said to contain one part scopolamine and 2 parts atropine.

- A mixture **may** have ingredients other than those mentioned in the wording of the ratio; generally they are inert and may be ignored if the mixture is not being weighed. However, if the mixture is being weighed to yield an amount having a specific quantity of a substance, all ingredients and their ratios must be known.

Using Ratios

A ratio may also be an expression of more than two substances in a mixture. A mixture containing 1 milligram hydrocodone, 120 milligrams acetaminophen and 100 milligrams lactose would be written as follows:

Hydrocodone: Acetaminophen: Lactose 1:120:100.

If 1 mg hydrocodone is present, this mixture would have a total weight of 1 + 120 + 100 = 221 mg.

Ratios have great utility in problem solving; therefore, their structures should be understood before progressing to proportion. Ratios may also be used to express quantities of a specific liquid in a mixture of liquids or solids in a liquid solution.

✍ CHECK YOUR UNDERSTANDING

1. Write the ratio of a solution containing 40 milligrams of drug in 1 milliliter of solution.

Answer: 40/1 or 40:1

2. Write the ratio of a solution containing 10 parts of an object liquid in 30 parts solvent.

Answer: 10:30 or 10/30

Caution: Sometimes, particularly when dealing with liquids, people will use the second part of the ratio (30 in the previous example) to denote the **total parts of solution** rather than the parts of solvent **in addition to** the parts of object liquid. This will become readily apparent when the student begins practice.

Proportion

According to *The American Heritage Dictionary*, proportion is defined as: "a relation between quantities such that if one varies, another varies as a multiple of the first."

The practical use of proportion lies with its ability to allow the technician to find an unknown amount of substance present in a known amount of mixture when given the ratio of substance to mixture. The technician is able to conduct calculations of this sort because of the concept of equivalence: that is, ratios may have different numbers and still be equal to each other. Thus, the ratios 2:1 and 4:2 are equivalent because the relative amounts of each substance in the ratio are the same.

The test for equivalency:

1. Multiply the number on the right of one ratio by the number on the left of the second ratio, and vice versa.
2. Compare the two answers found. If they are equal, the ratios are equivalent.

Example

Test the ratios 2:1 and 4:2 for equivalency:

a. $2 \times 2 = 4$, $1 \times 4 = 4$
b. Does 4 = 4? (Yes)
c. The ratios are equivalent.

This test also works when the ratios are expressed as fractions. Expressing the ratios as fractions tends to give most people a clearer visualization of what is occurring mathematically. It is suggested to the student that problems be set up this way.

The following example will be used since it is assumed that most students will already know the answer.

✍ CHECK YOUR UNDERSTANDING

There are 100 pennies in 1 dollar. How many pennies are in 3 dollars?

Technically speaking, the following is the correct way to set up the equation:

Equation # 1

$$\frac{100 \text{ pennies}}{x \text{ pennies}} = \frac{1 \text{ dollar}}{3 \text{ dollars}}$$

It should be done this way because 100 pennies = 1 dollar and x pennies equals 3 dollars. (A comparison of two equivalent ratios, 100:x and 1:3.)

To solve:

a. $100 \times 3 = 1 \times x$

b. $300 = X$

Answer: 300 pennies equal three dollars.

However, the goal of this text is to arrange equations so that problems may be solved quickly **and** accurately. For many people, arranging the equation in this manner increases both time expended to solve and the degree of inaccuracy incurred. So the following method is presented:

By rearranging the values, an equation is found that places the units where most of us have grown up thinking they belong:

Equation # 2

$$\frac{100 \text{ pennies}}{\text{dollar}} = \frac{x \text{ pennies}}{3 \text{ dollars}}$$

$$300 = x$$

Answer: 300 pennies = 3 dollars

Although this rearrangement may seem trivial, it becomes helpful when drug solutions with less familiar names than pennies and dollars are used. It **may** also be helpful to think of the dividing line shown between pennies and dollars as "per," e.g. 100 pennies "per" dollar = 100 pennies/dollar. One may substitute "in a" for "per" if this increases comfort.

✍ CHECK YOUR UNDERSTANDING

1. There are 10 milligrams of furosemide in 1 milliliter of furosemide injection. How many milligrams are contained in 10 milliliters?

Solution:

a. $\dfrac{10 \text{ mg}}{1 \text{ ml}} = \dfrac{x \text{ mg}}{10 \text{ ml}}$

b.   **Cross-multiply:** $10 \times 10 = 1 \times x$

c. $100 = X$

Answer: 100 milligrams

Note: The units involved are not multiplied by one another because ratios are being tested for equivalency.

Please also note the positioning of the units on both sides of the altered equation (equation # 2). When mg is placed in the numerator on one side of the equation, mg must also be placed in the numerator on the other side. This is not to say that mg must always be placed in the numerator, only that the unit's relative positions must be the same on both sides of the equation. However, if equation # 1 is used, mg will be in the numerator and denominator of one side, and ml would be on the other side of the equation.

2. *1 liter of drug solution contains 100 mg of drug. How many liters would it take to dispense a 500 mg dose?*

a. $\dfrac{100 \text{ mg}}{1 \text{ L}} = \dfrac{500 \text{ mg}}{x \text{ L}}$

b. **Cross-multiply:** 100x = 500

Answer: x = 5 Liters

Ratio and proportion have utility in problem solving in places other than the pharmacy.

3. *One ounce of cheese puffs contains 6 grams of fat. How many grams of fat are present in 5 ounces of cheese puffs?*

$\dfrac{6 \text{ grams}}{1 \text{ ounce}} = \dfrac{x \text{ grams}}{5 \text{ ounces}}$

Answer: x = 30 grams fat

❖ PRACTICE PROBLEMS FOR RATIO AND PROPORTION

Given the following equivalencies, solve the problems listed below:

$$1 \text{ inch} = 2.541 \text{ cm}$$
$$5280 \text{ feet} = 1 \text{ mile}$$
$$1 \text{ g fat} = 9 \text{ calories}$$
$$12 \text{ kopecs} = 1 \text{ dollar}$$

1. How many kopecs are in 5.5 dollars?
2. How many centimeters are in 2 yards? (**Hint:** Convert inches to centimeters.)
3. How many feet are in 6 miles?
4. A food contains 14 grams of fat. How many calories does the food supply as fat?
5. A solution of digoxin contains 50 mcg in each ml of solution. How many ml are required for a 125 mcg dose?
6. Dopamine injection solution contains 40 mg per ml. How many ml of dopamine are required if 400 mg are required to prepare an IV?
7. A solution of dobutamine containing 250 mg is required. How many ml of manufacturer-supplied dobutamine solution are required if each ml of solution contains 12.5 mg?
8. 10 ml of metoclopramide syrup contains 10 mg. How many ml are required for a 5 mg dose?
9. Amoxicillin is supplied as a suspension containing 125 mg per 5 ml. How many ml are needed for a 150 mg dose?
10. Dicloxacillin is supplied as a suspension containing 62.5 mg per 5 ml. How many ml are needed for the following (**Hint:** Find the total amount of drug needed before setting up the equation.)
    a. one 31.25 mg dose?
    b. one 125 mg dose?
    c. 10 doses of 125 mg each?
    d. 8 doses of 250 mg each?
11. A single shelf is able to contain 20 books the size of this text. If each book weighs 2 pounds, how many shelves are required for 90 books?
12. If a car should have its oil changed every 5,000 miles, how many oil changes are needed in 150,000 miles?

13. An office space is being rented according to its size. If the market rate is $2.70 per square foot, what would be the price if the office were 1500 square feet?
14. A cefazolin solution contains 100 mg per ml. What volume would be required for a 500 mg dose?
15. Each table ordered for a party will seat 10 guests. If there are to be 125 guests, how many tables will be needed?
16. One case of a drug will provide 70 doses. How many cases will be needed for 210 doses?
17. 105 Japanese yen are equivalent to one U.S. dollar. How many yen are needed to equal 75 dollars?
18. 10 milliliters of a solution contain 625 milligrams of drug. How many milligrams of drug are contained in one milliliter?
19. If it takes 5 trees to make one ton of paper, how many tons of paper can be made from 30 trees?
20. There are 3 grams of fat in 2 potato chips. How many grams of fat are in 6 chips?

Given ratios for the composition of the following mixtures, calculate how much of each ingredient is present:

21. 1 kg of 1:2 codeine: lactose
22. 500 g of 2:1 hydrocortisone: talc
23. 5 mg of 1:5 folic acid: sucrose
24. 100 g of 1:3 dinoprostone: surgilube
25. 4 pounds of 3:5 apples: oranges (Sometimes you *can* compare apples and oranges.)

Answer the following questions:

26. Are the ratios 3:5 and 2:9 equivalent?
27. Are the ratios of 5:9 and 10:18 equivalent?

Solve following problems using the formulas given in "Methods of Calculation":

28. Given 1 dollar = 100 pennies, solve the following:
    a. How many pennies in 18 dollars?
    b. How many dollars in 650 pennies?
    c. How many pennies in 9.5 dollars?
29. 2.14 English pounds = 1 dollar:
    a. How many pounds = 1500 dollars
    b. How many dollars = 214 pounds
30. A car can travel 50 miles in 1 hour. How many miles can be traveled in 3 hours?

Chapter 14
ROUNDING

In this chapter:
- *Rules of Rounding*

RULES OF ROUNDING

You may find that the absolute answer to a problem will be many decimal places in length. Because of the sensitivity requirements of the various measuring devices in commercial use, expression of decimals beyond two decimal places is unnecessary most of the time.

When the measuring device is too insensitive to measure the number of decimal places found in the final calculation, the answer should be rounded.

Points to Remember

- When the number occupying the decimal one space to the right of the decimal to be rounded is ≥ 5, the decimal is rounded up.
    - i.e. Round 0.015 to two decimal places.
    - **Answer:** 0.02
- When the number occupying the decimal one space to the right of the decimal to be rounded is < 5, the decimal is rounded down.
    - i.e. Round 0.014 to two decimal places.
    - **Answer:** 0.01

❖ PRACTICE PROBLEMS

1. Round 0.1235 to three decimal places.
2. Round 0.263 to two decimal places.
3. Round 0.712 to one decimal place.
4. Round 1.614 to two decimal places.
5. Round 2.7778 to three decimal places.
6. Round 1.25167 to three decimal places.
7. Round 0.862 to two decimal places.
8. Round 0.12345678 to two decimal places.
9. Round 1.357 to one decimal place.
10. Round 127.1892 to three decimal places.

Round the following:

11. 1.356 to 2 decimal places
12. 50.13579 to 1 decimal place
13. 5.246810 to 4 decimal places
14. 2.1711 to 3 decimal places
15. 3.918 to 2 decimal places

Chapter 15
DOSING

In this chapter:
- *Body Surface Area Dosing*
- *Dosing of Tablets and Capsules*
- *Dispensing Various Dosage Forms*
- *Dosing Constant Infusions*

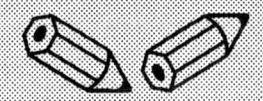

DEFINING DOSING

For a drug to exert its effect beneficially on the patient, the amount given must be controlled. The amount of drug given to a patient is known as the dose. Too much drug, and the patient may experience serious adverse effects; too little drug, and the patient will not derive any benefit. Therefore, it is important for the pharmacy technician to know how to measure, count, or otherwise dispense the proper dose to the patient. Even though the pharmacy technician's work will be checked by a pharmacist before leaving the pharmacy, the patient is best served by both technician and pharmacist paying close attention to the delivery of the correct dose.

The optimal dose of a drug in this country is determined through clinical studies done during the process of obtaining marketing approval from the Food and Drug Administration. However, new doses are sometimes determined after the approval process is completed, most frequently for uses for which the drug was not initially approved.

Points to Remember

There are many ways a drug may be dosed:
- As a standard dose that everyone receives regardless of age, weight, height, sex or disease
- By the patient weight
- By disease state
- By kidney or other organ function

- By the amount of body surface area the patient has
- The most common way is to determine the dose based on the patient's weight. The dose will generally be given in milligrams of drug per kilogram of body weight, or mg/kg.

To determine the dose of a drug for a patient when the literature states that the drug is to be dosed in mg/kg:

$$\text{Patient weight (kg)} \times \frac{mg}{kg} \text{ (dose)}$$

CHECK YOUR UNDERSTANDING

1. One possible dose for ondansetron is 0.15 mg/kg. If a patient weighs 70 kilograms, what will the dose be for the patient?

Solution:

$$70 \text{ kg} \times \frac{0.15 \text{ mg}}{kg} = 10.5 \text{ mg}$$

Answer: 10.5 mg

2. A patient weighs 100 kilograms. What will the patient's dose be if gentamicin 2 mg/kg is to be given?

Solution:

$$100 \text{ kg} \times \frac{2 \text{ mg}}{kg} = 200 \text{ mg}$$

Answer: 200 mg

Dosage Range

Very commonly, a drug will have a variety of doses that may be used. The correct dose to be chosen depends on such patient variables as patient disease, severity of disease, and organ function. The variety of dosages that may be used for a particular drug is known as the **dosage range**. Any dose desired that is within dosage range will be safe for most people. However, as the dose increases, so does the likelihood of adverse effects caused by the drug.

An example of dosage range is "High-dose metoclopramide for chemotherapy-induced emesis" 1-2 mg/kg. Obviously, this dosage range applies to chemotherapy-induced emesis; it would not be appropriate for most uses of metoclopramide. The range provided infers that any dose between 1 and 2 mg/kg is appropriate for this treatment.

To determine if a dose to be given falls into the dosage range:

$$\frac{\text{dose (mg)}}{\text{weight (kg)}} = \text{dose/kg to be compared to the dosage range}$$

CHECK YOUR UNDERSTANDING

A 75 mg dose of metoclopramide is ordered for a chemotherapy-induced emesis. The dosage range for this indication is 1-2 mg/kg. Is this dose appropriate for a 50 kg patient?

Solution:

a: $\dfrac{75 \text{ (mg)}}{50 \text{ (kg)}} = \dfrac{1.5 \text{ (mg)}}{kg}$

b: Compare the answer (1.5 mg/kg) with the dosage range (1-2 mg/kg).

Answer: Yes, the dose is appropriate.

BODY SURFACE AREA DOSING

Another method of calculating appropriate dosing of medications is the Body Surface Area method (BSA). This method utilizes the total volume a person's body displaces rather than patient weight. This method is used most commonly in dosing medications used to destroy tumors.

BSA is measured in square meters (m^2), and dosing is measured in mg/m^2.

A patient's BSA is found by utilizing the chart found on the following pages. To read the chart accurately, use a straight edge to line up the patient's height and the patient's weight. By following a line drawn between these two points on the chart (referred to as a nomogram), the patient's BSA is determined. See the Adult Body Surface Area Dosing Chart on page 106 and the Children's Body Surface Area Dosing Chart on page 107.

Because the tables are based upon height and weight only, not age, an adult who possessed a height and weight smaller than that found on the adult charts could have his or her BSA determined by the table meant for children.

The calculation of drug dose based on BSA is carried out in much the same way as the mg/kg method.

BSA Equation

$$\text{BSA (m}^2\text{)} \times \text{mg/m}^2 = \text{dose}$$

✍ CHECK YOUR UNDERSTANDING

1. An adult is five feet, five inches in height and 200 pounds in weight. What is the patient's BSA?

Solution:

a. Convert 5 feet, 5 inches (5 feet $\times \frac{12 \text{ inches}}{\text{foot}}$) + 5 inches = 65 inches

b. Using a straight edge, such as a ruler, locate 65 inches in the "height" column found at the far left.

c. Next, keeping one end of the straight edge on 65 inches, locate 200 pounds in the "weight" column found at the far right.

d. The value underlined by the straight edge in the "body surface" column (center) is, quite obviously, the patient's BSA. In this case, the answer is 1.98 m^2 (not quite 1.98, but the nomogram does not allow for greater accuracy).

2. A child weighs 10 kg and is 70 cm in height. What is the child's BSA?

Solution:

a. Locate 70 cm in the "height" column.

b. Locate 10 kg in the "weight" column.

c. Follow the straight edge to the middle "body surface" column.

d. The value found is 0.415 (the straight edge lies in between 0.41 and 0.42).

3. A patient has a BSA of 1.5 m^2 and is to receive a dose of 40 mg/m^2. Calculate the dose for this patient.

Solution:

1.5 m^2 × 40 mg/m^2 = 60 mg dose

Answer: 60 mg dose

Adult Body Surface Area Dosing Chart

Nomogram for determination of body surface from height and mass[1]

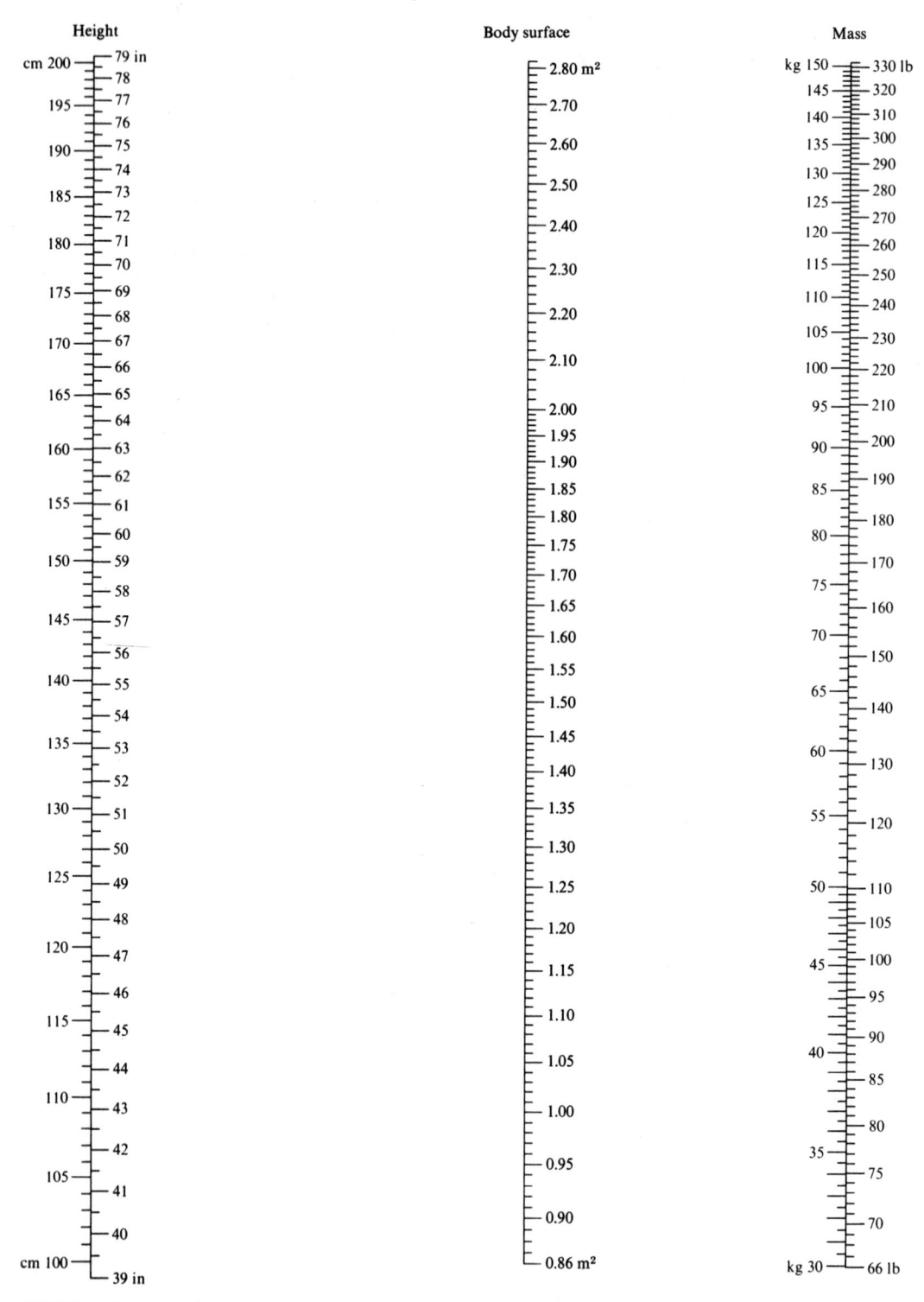

Height	Body surface	Mass
cm 200 — 79 in ... cm 100 — 39 in	2.80 m² ... 0.86 m²	kg 150 — 330 lb ... kg 30 — 66 lb

[1] From the formula of Du Bois and Du Bois, *Arch. intern. Med.*, **17**, 863 (1916): $S = M^{0.425} \times H^{0.725} \times 71.84$, or $\log S = \log M \times 0.425 + \log H \times 0.725 + 1.8564$ (S: body surface in cm², M: mass in kg, H: height in cm).

C. Lentner (Ed.) *Geigy Scientific Tables.* 8th edition, volume 1, Ciba-Geigy, Basle, 1981. pp. 226-227. Reprinted by permission of CIBA.

Children's Body Surface Area Dosing Chart

Nomogram for determination of body surface from height and mass[1]

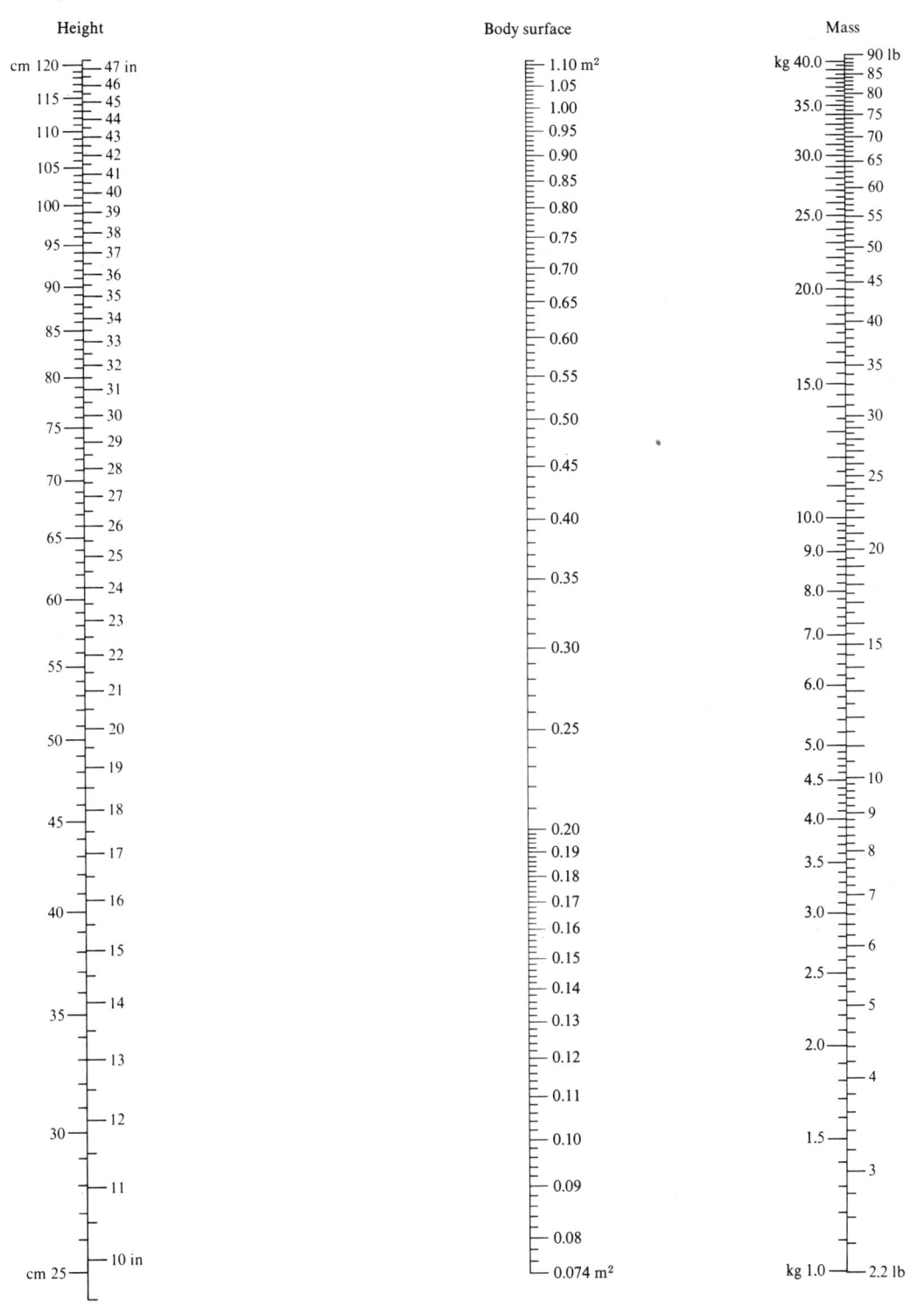

Height	Body surface	Mass
cm 120 — 47 in ... cm 25 — 10 in	1.10 m² ... 0.074 m²	kg 40.0 — 90 lb ... kg 1.0 — 2.2 lb

[1] From the formula of Du Bois and Du Bois, *Arch. intern. Med.*, **17**, 863 (1916): $S = M^{0.425} \times H^{0.725} \times 71.84$, or $\log S = \log M \times 0.425 + \log H \times 0.725 + 1.8564$ (S: body surface in cm², M: mass in kg, H: height in cm).

C. Lentner (Ed.) *Geigy Scientific Tables*. 8th edition, volume 1, Ciba-Geigy, Basle, 1981. pp. 226-227. Reprinted by permission of CIBA.

DOSING OF TABLETS AND CAPSULES

The most common dosage forms are tablets and capsules. Usually, a prescription will order a dose of one tablet or capsule. However, there will be times when a dose larger than the largest tablet or capsule available will be required. When these situations occur, a simple calculation may be employed.

To determine the number of tablets or capsules needed for a dose, use the following formula:

# of capsules or tablets to dispense = dose needed ÷ quantity of each tablet or capsule

or

$$\text{dose (mg)} \times \frac{1 \text{ tablet or capsule}}{\text{quantity in each tablet or capsule}} = \text{number of capsules or tablets}$$

DOSING OF LIQUIDS

When a patient can tolerate the oral route but is unable to swallow a tablet or capsule, a liquid dosage form may be used. Small children and patients who have suffered strokes most often receive oral medications in liquid form. Psychiatric patients may receive liquid dosage forms when it has been determined that the patient is not swallowing the tablet or capsule but is hiding it under the tongue instead so that he or she spit it out unobserved. Additionally, liquid dosage forms are used to prevent psychiatric patients from hoarding medication for a suicide attempt. In these cases, administration of the liquid dosage form assures that the patient is taking the medication.

To measure liquid doses correctly, one must understand the concept of concentration. **Concentration** refers to the volume or weight of a target substance contained in a specific volume of drug solution. The weight is normally measured in milligrams and the volume is most often either for each milliliter or 5 milliliters (teaspoonsful) of preparation. This is expressed verbally as "mg per ml," "mg per 5 ml," or "mg per teaspoon," and written mg/ml, mg/5 ml and mg/tsp.

To determine volume to dispense using the dose needed and the concentration:

Volume needed for dose = dose needed ÷ concentration

or

dose × ml/mg = volume needed

✍ CHECK YOUR UNDERSTANDING

The following problems will test your ability to dose tablets/capsules and liquids.

1. A 500 mg dose is needed. How many 250 mg tablets will satisfy this dose?

Solution:

a.   # of tablets to dispense = 500 ÷ 250 → 2 tablets

  or

b. $500 \text{ mg} \times \frac{1 \text{ tab}}{250 \text{ mg}} = \frac{500}{250}$ tab or 2 tablets

Answer: 2 tablets

2. Haloperidol is available in a concentration of 2 mg/ml. How many ml are needed for a 3mg dose?

a.   Volume needed = $3 \text{ mg} \div \frac{2 \text{ mg}}{1 \text{ ml}}$ or $3 \text{ mg} \times \frac{1 \text{ ml}}{2 \text{ mg}} = \frac{3}{2}$ ml or 1.5 ml

or

b. $3 \text{ mg} \times \dfrac{1 \text{ ml}}{2 \text{ mg}} = \dfrac{3}{2}$ or 1.5 ml

Answer: 1.5 ml

(The above example shows that dividing by a fraction is the same as multiplying by a reciprocal of that same fraction.)

Once the technician has become accustomed to doing this the long way, he or she may use a shortcut utilizing the above example:

Volume needed = $3 \div 2 = \dfrac{3}{2}$ or $1\dfrac{1}{2}$ ml

Caution: Do not use the shortcut until you understand why it works.

Why It Works

After examining the first example, one finds that all the units cancel out except ml, which finds its way into the answer. Since this cancellation of units will always occur, the shortcut drops them from the very beginning.

This method also works when the concentration is given as mg/tsp, with the following difference: the answer is in the number of teaspoons instead of ml. This is an important point because obviously 1 ½ teaspoons is not the same as 1 ½ ml.

✍ CHECK YOUR UNDERSTANDING

1. Amoxicillin suspension is available as a concentration of 125 mg/teaspoonful. How many teaspoons are needed for a 150 mg dose?

Solution:

a. Volume needed = $150 \text{ mg} \div \dfrac{125 \text{ mg}}{\text{tsp}}$ or $150 \text{ mg} \times \dfrac{\text{tsp}}{125 \text{ mg}} \rightarrow 1\dfrac{1}{5}$ tsp

or

b. **Shortcut:** $150 \div 125 = 1\dfrac{25}{150}$ or $1\dfrac{1}{5}$ tsp

Answer: $1\dfrac{1}{5}$ tsp

Since 1 ⅕ teaspoons is cumbersome, if not impossible to measure using traditionally calibrated oral liquid syringes, it is more appropriate to convert teaspoons to milliliters: 1 teaspoon = 5 ml.

Utilizing the previous example:

To convert: $x \text{ teaspoons} \times \dfrac{5 \text{ ml}}{\text{teaspoon}} = x \text{ ml}$

$\dfrac{6}{5} \text{ teaspoons} \times \dfrac{5 \text{ ml}}{\text{teaspoon}} = \dfrac{30}{5}$ or 6 ml

The following shortcut may not seem short initially, but it does make life easier and is actually quicker once it is understood:

Step 1: Convert concentration from mg/tsp to mg/ml by dividing mg/tsp by 5 (5ml = 1 teaspoon)

Step 2: Divide dose needed by concentration/ml

110 Dosing

2. Ampicillin suspension is available as a 250 mg/teaspoonful preparation. How many ml are needed for a 50 mg dose?

Step 1: $\dfrac{250 \text{ mg}}{5 \text{ ml}}$ or → 250 ÷ 5 → $\dfrac{50 \text{ mg}}{\text{ml}}$

Step 2: $\dfrac{\text{(dose)} \div \text{(conc)}}{50 \div 50} = 1 \text{ml}$

Using Proportion

a. $\dfrac{250 \text{ mg}}{5 \text{ ml}} = \dfrac{50 \text{ mg}}{x \text{ ml}}$ or $\dfrac{250 \text{ mg}}{50 \text{ mg}} = \dfrac{5 \text{ ml}}{x \text{ ml}}$

b. Cross multiply: 250 x = 250

c. Solve: $\dfrac{250x}{250} = \rightarrow x = 1 \text{ml}$

Answer: x = 1 ml

3. Furosemide is available in a concentration of 10 mg/ml. A 20 mg dose is needed. What volume must be dispensed? (Use proportion.)

a. $\dfrac{10 \text{ mg}}{1 \text{ ml}} = \dfrac{20 \text{ mg}}{x \text{ ml}}$ or $\dfrac{10 \text{ mg}}{20 \text{ mg}} = \dfrac{1 \text{ ml}}{x \text{ ml}}$

b. 10 x = 20   10 x = 20

Answer: x = 2 ml

It is important to understand how to solve concentration problems as there are a multitude of vastly different concentrations used for liquid drug products.

Some commercially available liquid drug products and their concentrations are provided in the following table:

Some Common Liquid Drug Products and Their Concentrations

Drug	Concentration
Furosemide oral solution	10 mg/ml
Digoxin elixir	0.05 mg/ml
Haloperidol concentrate	2 mg/ml
Aminophylline oral solution	105 mg/5ml
Fluphenazine elixir	0.5 mg/ml
Diphenhydramine elixir	12.5 mg/5ml
Metoclopramide syrup	1 mg/ml
Ranitidine syrup	15 mg/ml
Dexamethasone elixir	0.5 mg/5ml
Dexamethasone oral solution	1 mg/ml

As the above table illustrates, there are a wide variety of concentrations utilized by manufacturers. Some reasons for these differing concentrations are:

1. **Physical**—Some drugs are not very soluble, and, thus, their concentrations must be kept low to keep the drugs in solution.
2. **Practical**—Many drugs may be highly soluble, but their normal doses are small, so the concentration is set at a low value that allows the dose to be measured easily. Conversely, some drugs are dispensed in higher doses; therefore, they are made more concentrated. This allows the dose to be presented to the patient in a convenient volume. Many drugs are made available in several concentrations because of the wide dosage ranges employed.

Because of the above-mentioned variables, one should always read the label and determine the concentration of the liquid dose form before measuring the dose.

DISPENSING THE VARIOUS DOSAGE FORMS

In the majority of situations, a patient will present a complete prescription for dispensing. However, sometimes a measure of reasoning will need to be employed to determine the quantity of the drug to be dispensed. Often a physician will write for a specific dose to be taken with a given frequency for a specified number of days but will omit the quantity to dispense. In this instance, the following formula may be employed:

$$\frac{\text{number of caps or tabs}}{\text{dose}} \times \frac{\text{doses}}{\text{day}} \times \text{days of therapy} = \text{number of capsules or tablets to complete therapy}$$

✍ CHECK YOUR UNDERSTANDING

1. You are presented with the following prescription. How many capsules are needed for the therapy?

Amoxicillin 250 mg caps

$\frac{\cdot}{\text{I}}$ t.i.d. × 10 days

a. The $\frac{\cdot}{\text{I}}$ signifies the number of capsules per dose where $\frac{\cdot}{\text{I}}$ = 1. Physicians often write numerals this way; the dots should be in the same quantity as the marks below, i.e. $\frac{\cdot\cdot}{\text{II}}$ = 2, $\frac{\cdot\cdot\cdot}{\text{III}}$ = 3, etc. This can be helpful as it prevents a 2 from being confused with a 7.

b. T.i.d. indicates the frequency with which the patient will take medication. T.i.d. is an abbreviation for three times daily (see Chapter 1, "The Language of Pharmacy.")

c. × 10 days—the patient will take the medication for ten days.

d. $\frac{1 \text{ cap}}{\text{dose}} \times \frac{3 \text{ doses}}{\text{day}} \times 10 \text{ days} = 30 \text{ caps}$

Answer: 30 capsules will be dispensed.

This formula also works for liquid medications; however, the concentrations of the liquid must be considered. This may be accomplished in one of two ways:

1. Determine the total quantity of drug the patient will take for the course of therapy; then divide by the concentration to find the volume to dispense.

   or

2. Determine the volume of each dose; then, substitute this volume into the formula in place of the number of tablets or capsules per dose.

112 Dosing

Amoxicillin 250 mg/5 ml

$\frac{1}{2}$ tsp t.i.d. × 10 days

Solution:

Using Method # 1

a. 1 tsp = 5 ml **so** $\frac{1}{2}$ tsp = 2.5 ml

b. Find out how many mg of Amoxicillin are in $\frac{1}{2}$ tsp using the method most comfortable for the technician:

Using Proportion

$$\frac{250 \text{ mg}}{5 \text{ ml}} = \frac{x \text{ mg}}{2.5 \text{ ml}}$$

$$5x = 625$$

$$x = 125 \text{ mg}$$

c. $\frac{125 \text{ mg}}{\text{dose}} \times \frac{3 \text{ doses}}{\text{day}} \times 10 \text{ days} \div \frac{250 \text{ mg}}{5 \text{ ml}}$

or

$\frac{125 \text{ mg}}{\text{dose}} \times \frac{3 \text{ doses}}{\text{day}} \times 10 \text{ days} \times \frac{5 \text{ ml}}{250 \text{ mg}} = \frac{18750 \text{ ml}}{250}$

$\downarrow$

75

Answer: 75 ml are needed for 10 days of therapy

Solution:

Using Method #2

a. 1 tsp. = 5 ml **so** $\frac{1}{2}$ tsp. = 2.5 ml

b. $\frac{2.5 \text{ ml}}{\text{dose}} \times \frac{3 \text{ doses}}{\text{day}} \times 10 \text{ days} = 75 \text{ ml}$

Answer: 75 ml are needed to complete a 10-day therapy.

CONSTANT INFUSIONS

Many drugs are given by continuous intravenous infusions rather than large infrequent doses. This is done primarily for the following reasons:

1. The drug's effect does not last long enough to allow any time to pass in between doses.
2. A drug exhibits wide variations in effect and clearance from the body based on numerous individual patient variations.
3. The patient will experience rapidly changing dose requirements and more or less drug will be immediately required.

Drugs Requiring Constant Infusions

Vecuronium

This drug is used to paralyze patients while a machine breathes for them. It requires a constant infusion in this setting because of its short duration and the need to keep the patient fully paralyzed.

Aminophylline

Used to keep the passageways of the lungs open, this drug is very toxic if allowed to accumulate. Multiple individual variances cause this drug to be difficult to dose properly when the patient needs it most. Blood levels of the drug are drawn periodically, and the infusion rate is changed based on the results of those tests.

Nitroglycerin

This drug is used to keep blood flowing into the arteries and veins that feed oxygen to the heart. The amount is related to the amount of chest pain the patient has. Initially, the patient may require large amounts. As time progresses, these needs become less, and the infusion is slowed until it is no longer needed.

Dosing Constant Infusions

Depending on the institution preference and the technician laws of various states, the technician may determine how quickly the infusion is to flow. Therefore, it is important to understand how these rates are determined.

Some infusions are dosed utilizing a specific amount of drug for each unit of body weight that the patient will receive in a specific period of time. For instance, if the specific amount of drug is 1 mg, the unit of body weight is 1 kg, and the specific period of time is 1 minute, the dose would be written as:

$$1 mg/kg/min \text{ or } 1 \text{ mg Kg}^{-1} \text{ min}^{-1}$$

and expressed verbally as:

"one milligram per kilogram per minute"

Other infusions do not employ body weight in the determination of their doses. Such infusions normally will have the rate stated as mg/min (milligrams per minute).

In order to calculate the infusion rate, the concentration of the solution at hand is also required. Many times this concentration will need to be converted from mg/ml to mcg/ml so **be careful!**

Once all of the above information has been collected, the following formula may be used:

$$\text{infusion rate} = \frac{\text{dose}}{\text{min}} \times \frac{60 \text{ min}}{\text{hr}} \div \text{concentration}$$

and

concentration can be mg/ml or mcg/ml

✍ CHECK YOUR UNDERSTANDING

1. *A 10 kg patient is to receive a drug at a rate of 1mg/kg/min. If the drug solution has a concentration of 1000 mg/100 ml, what will the infusion rate be in ml/hr?*

   a. *Important Facts*
   wt: 10 kg
   dose: 1 mg/kg/min

114 Dosing

  concentration: 1000 mg/100ml (10 mg/ml may also be used since it is equivalent to 1000 mg/100 ml)

b. $\dfrac{\text{dose}}{\text{min}} \times \dfrac{60 \text{ min}}{\text{hr}} \div \text{concentration} = \text{infusion rate}$

  $10 \text{kg} \times \dfrac{1 \text{ mg}}{\text{kg} \cdot \text{min}} \times \dfrac{60 \text{ min}}{\text{hour}} \div \dfrac{10 \text{ mg}}{\text{ml}}$

  $10 \text{ kg} \times \dfrac{1 \text{ mg}}{\text{kg} \cdot \text{min}} \times \dfrac{60 \text{ min}}{\text{hour}} \times \dfrac{\text{ml}}{10 \text{ mg}} = \dfrac{600 \text{ ml}}{10 \text{ hr}} \rightarrow \dfrac{60 \text{ ml}}{\text{hr}}$

Answer: Infusion rate = 60 ml/hr

2. *A patient is to receive a drug infusion at 2 mg/min. The concentration of the solution is 1000 mg/250 ml and the patient weighs 60 kg. What is the rate in ml/hr?*

a. **Important Facts**

  wt: not needed

  dose: 2mg/min

  concentration: 1000 mg/250 ml or 4mg/ml

b. $\dfrac{\text{dose}}{\text{min}} \times \dfrac{60 \text{min}}{\text{hr}} \div \text{concentration} = \text{infusion rate}$

  $\dfrac{2 \text{ mg}}{\text{min}} \times \dfrac{60 \text{ min}}{\text{hr}} \div \dfrac{4 \text{ mg}}{\text{ml}}$

  $\dfrac{2 \text{ mg}}{\text{ml}} \times \dfrac{60 \text{ min}}{\text{hr}} \times \dfrac{\text{ml}}{4 \text{ mg}} = \dfrac{120 \text{ml}}{4 \text{hr}} \rightarrow \dfrac{30 \text{ml}}{\text{hr}}$

Answer: Infusion rate = 30 ml/hr

3. *A 100 kg patient is to receive a dopamine infusion at the rate of 4 mcg/kg/min. If the infusion has a concentration of 400mg/250ml, what will the rate be in ml/hr?*

a. **Important Facts**

  wt: 100 kg

  dose: 4 mcg/kg/min

  concentration: 400 mg/250 ml (This must be converted to 400,000 mcg/250 ml or 1600 mcg/ml before calculations are done.)

b. $100 \text{ kg} \times \dfrac{4 \text{ mcg}}{\text{kg} \cdot \text{min}} \times \dfrac{60 \text{ min}}{\text{hr}} \times \dfrac{\text{ml}}{1,600 \text{ mcg}} = \dfrac{24,000 \text{ ml}}{1,600 \text{ hr}}$

  $\downarrow$

  15 ml/hr

Answer: The infusion must be run at a rate of 15 ml/hr.

As the preceding examples show, the calculation of constant infusions is merely a fusion of the dosing calculations learned previously.

These infusions deliver a dose (mcg/kg) over a shorter period of time (every minute instead of t.i.d.) than that described in earlier sections, but the calculation and concept are still the same. The dose to be delivered is converted to volume in the same way as earlier liquid drug product problems.

CALCULATING FLOW RATES USING DROP FACTORS

After an infusion rate has been calculated, it must be delivered to the patient. This is done most commonly by one of two ways:

1. By infusion pump, whereby the nurse will enter the infusion rate into a pump that is connected to the IV bag. This pump will then very accurately control the infusion rate.

   or

2. By using an infusion set with a calibrated drip chamber. These infusion sets have a portion of their tubing that is larger than the rest of the infusion set. The liquid from the IV bag drips down into this widened area at a rate that is controlled by gravity and an adjustable restrictive device. The nurse can control how fast the IV flows by raising or lowering the bag or by loosening or tightening the restrictive device. Obviously, there are no calculations involved using the pump; one has only to press the buttons correctly. The drip chamber, however, requires observation and calculation. The drip chamber is calibrated to deliver one milliliter of fluid by dripping a certain number of drops into the chamber. The package will state this drop factor on the package as drops/ml. If the set states on its packaging "10 drops/ml", then 10 drops falling into the chamber will deliver one milliliter of fluid to the patient. This drop factor is used to convert **ml/hr** to **drops/min** so that the nurse can adjust the flow rate properly.

The following formula is used:

$$\text{drops/min} = \frac{\text{ml}}{\text{hr}} \times \frac{\text{drops}}{\text{ml}} \times \frac{1 \text{ hr}}{60 \text{ min}}$$

✍ CHECK YOUR UNDERSTANDING

1. An IV is to flow at the rate of 60 ml/hr. If the infusion set has a drop factor of 10 drops/ml what is the rate in drops/min?

Solution:

a. $\dfrac{\text{drops}}{\text{min}} = \dfrac{60 \text{ ml}}{\text{hr}} \times \dfrac{10 \text{ drops}}{\text{ml}} \times \dfrac{1 \text{ hr}}{60 \text{ min}} \rightarrow \dfrac{600 \text{ drops}}{60 \text{ min}} \downarrow \dfrac{10 \text{ drops}}{\text{min}}$

Answer: 10 drops/min = 60 ml/hr

2. An IV is to be infused at a rate of 120 ml/hr. If the infusion set has a drop factor of 15 drops/ml, what is the rate in drops/min?

Solution:

$\dfrac{\text{drops}}{\text{min}} = \dfrac{120 \text{ ml}}{\text{hr}} \times \dfrac{15 \text{ drops}}{\text{ml}} \times \dfrac{1 \text{ hr}}{60 \text{ min}} \rightarrow \dfrac{1800 \text{ drops}}{60 \text{ min}} \downarrow \dfrac{30 \text{ drops}}{\text{min}}$

Answer: $\dfrac{30 \text{ drops}}{\text{min}} = \dfrac{120 \text{ ml}}{\text{hr}}$

After doing this calculation, the nurse will start the infusion and count drops. Most nurses will not count for a whole minute but rather for 15 or 30 seconds. Consequently, if 120 ml/hr = 30 drops/min, and the nurse counts for only 30 seconds, then the number of drops corresponding to 120 ml/hr will be less. Thus, the following calculation is used:

$$\frac{30 \text{ drops}}{60 \text{ seconds}} = \frac{x \text{ drops}}{30 \text{ seconds}} \rightarrow 60x = 900$$

$$x = 15 \text{ drops}$$

Therefore, if the nurse counts for 30 seconds and 15 drops fall, the correct rate has been achieved. If either too few or too many drops are falling, the IV bag will be raised to increase the rate, or lowered to decrease it, or the constricting clamp will be used to regulate the flow.

CALCULATING INFUSION RATES BASED ON HANG TIME

Often, a patient requires only a certain amount of fluid given over a short period of time to meet his or her fluid requirements. This is frequently the case when drugs are given intravenously; some drugs must be diluted in a certain amount of volume and given over a certain period of time to avoid toxicity. Another example is a technique called **fluid bolusing**. This technique delivers an amount of electrolyte solution over a period of several hours and is used to replace electrolytes needed by the patient.

On both examples, the infusion runs for a short period of time, then stops. To calculate the rate at which these infusions are to run, the following formula is used:

$$\frac{\text{volume to infuse}}{\text{time of infusion}} = \text{rate of infusion}$$

✍ CHECK YOUR UNDERSTANDING

1. *A patient is to receive a bolus of 500 ml of 3% saline to correct a sodium imbalance. If the infusion is to run over 4 hours, what is the rate in ml/hr? (After doing this calculation, the health care provider will know how to set his pump or administration set in order to deliver the fluid over a specified period of time.)*

Solution:

$$\frac{500 \text{ ml}}{4 \text{ hours}} = \frac{125 \text{ ml}}{\text{hr}}$$

Answer: The solution must be run at 125 ml/hr for 4 hours.

2. *A patient is to receive a 2 liter bolus of D₅W to correct dehydration. What will the rate be in ml/hr if the bolus is to infuse over 8 hours?*

Solution:

$$2 \text{ L} = \frac{2000 \text{ ml}}{8 \text{ hours}} = \frac{250 \text{ ml}}{\text{hour}}$$

Answer: The infusion must run at 250 ml/hr for 8 hour

❖ PRACTICE PROBLEMS

Given the following liquid drug products and their concentrations:

        Haloperidol Concentrate—2 mg/ml

        Furosemide Elixir—10 mg/ml

        Digoxin Elixir—50 mcg/ml

        Fluphenazine Elixir—0.5 mg/ml

        Amoxicillin Susp—250 mg/5ml

        Dicloxacillin Susp—62.5 mg/5 ml

        Cefixime Susp—100 mg/5 ml

        Nafcillin Inj—250 mg/ml

        Dexamethasone Inj—4 mg/ml

State the volume needed to dispense the following drug doses:

1. Dexamethasone 10 mg
2. Haloperidol concentrate 10 mg
3. A 150 mg dose of cefixime
4. Nafcillin Inj 500 mg
5. Furosemide 40 mg
6. Digoxin 0.75 mg
7. Fluphenazine 5 mg
8. Amoxicillin 500 mg
9. Dicloxacillin 250 mg
10. Cefixime 400 mg
11. Haloperidol 4 mg
12. Digoxin 0.125 mg
13. Fluphenazine 2.5 mg
14. Dicloxacillin 125 mg
15. Furosemide 30 mg
16. Nafcillin 250 mg
17. Dexamethasone 1 mg
18. Amoxicillin 125 mg

Based on the patient BSA and mg/m² dose, calculate the amount of drug needed for each dose:

	BSA	mg/m²
19.	2m²	35
20.	1.75m²	40
21.	2.12m²	50

An initial dose of gentamicin 2 mg/kg is to be given to the following patients. Calculate each patient's dose based on his/her weight:

22. 70 kg
23. 90 kg
24. 68 kg
25. 210 pounds
26. 101 kg
27. A dose of fluphenazine 5 mg is needed, but your pharmacy stocks only 1 mg tabs. How 1 mg tabs are needed?
28. Calculate the number of 0.5 haloperidol tablets needed for a 1.5 mg dose.
29. A prescription is written for metronidazole 500 mg b.i.d. × 10 days. You have 250 mg tablets only. How many of these tablets are required to complete therapy?

118 Dosing

30. *Solve the following problem:*

    Penicillin solution 250 mg/5 ml $\frac{1}{1}$ tsp q.i.d. × 7 days. How many ml will be needed to complete therapy?

31. A constant infusion of dobutamine is to be given to a 70 kg patient. The infusion has a concentration of 500 mg/250 ml. If the patient is to receive 5 mcg/kg/min, what is the rate in ml/hr?

32. A dopamine infusion having a concentration of 400 mg/250ml is to be delivered to a patient at the rate of 6 mcg/kg/min. If the patient weighs 80 kg, what will the rate of the infusion be in ml/hr?

33. Lidocaine is to be given to a 100 kg patient at a rate of 2 mg/min. If the concentration of the infusion is 2 g/500 ml, what is the rate in ml/hr?

34. *Given the following prescription:* Haloperidol concentrate 2 mg/ml 5 mg b.i.d. × 30 days. How many ml will be dispensed?

35. An IV is to be infused at a rate of 150 ml/hr. If the infusion set has a drop factor of 10 drops/ml, what is the rate in drops/min?

36. An IV is to be infused at 125 ml/hr. If the drop factor of the infusion set is 15 drops/ml, what is the rate in drops/min?

37. A dose of gentamicin must be given over 1 hour to avoid toxicity. If the dose of gentamicin is diluted to a total volume of 100 ml, what will the rate of infusion have to be to deliver the dose over 1 hour?

38. A fluid bolus is to be given to a patient. If the bolus has a total volume of 500 ml and is to run over 2 hours, what must the rate be in ml/hr?

Given the following drug strengths:

> *Reglan—10 mg tablets*
> *Bumex—0.5 mg tablets*
> *Propylthiouracil—50 mg tablets*
> *Digoxin—0.125 mg tablets*

Calculate the amount of tablets per dose:

39. Reglan 30 mg
40. Bumex 2 mg
41. Propylthiouracil 250 mg
42. Digoxin 0.375 mg
43. Reglan 50 mg
44. Bumex 1.5 mg
45. Propylthiouracil 150 mg
46. Digoxin 0.0625 mg

Given the following liquid dose forms:

> *Amoxcillin 125 mg/5 ml*
> *Penicillin VK 250 mg/5 ml*
> *Dicloxacillin 62.5 mg/5 ml*
> *Ferrous sulfate 220 mg/5 ml*
> *Furosemide 10 mg/ ml*

Calculate the volume needed for the following doses:

47.	Amoxicillin 250 mg	48.	Amoxicillin 62.5 mg
49.	Amoxicillin 150 mg	50.	Penicillin 125 mg
51.	Penicillin 300 mg	52.	Dicloxicillin 125 mg
53.	Dicloxicillin 31.25 mg	54.	Ferrous sulfate 110 mg
55.	Ferrous sulfate 132 mg	56.	Furosemide 1 mg
57.	Furosemide 5 mg	58.	Furosemide 15 mg

Given patient weight and dose/kg, calculate the dose needed for that patient:

	Weight	Dose
59.	60 kg	2 mg/kg
60.	180 lbs	0.15 mg/kg
61.	90 kg	40 mg/kg
62.	110 kg	20 mg/kg
63.	85 kg	0.1 mg/kg

Given the drugs' dosing range below, determine whether or not the following doses are appropriate:

>Gentamicin 1-2 mg/kg
>Digoxin 2-4 mcg/kg
>Acetaminophen 10-15 mg/kg

	Drug	Dose	Patient Weight
64.	Digoxin	0.25 mg	100 kg
65.	Digoxin	0.25 mg	60 kg
66.	Acetaminophen	1,000 mg	70 kg
67.	Gentamicin	120 mg	70 kg
68.	Gentamicin	200 mg	90 kg

69. Vincristine is to be given as a dose of 1 mg/m^2. If the patient has a BSA of 1.5 m^2, what is the dose?

70. Given a BSA of 2 m^2, what size dose would be given to a patient requiring a 40 mg/m^2 dose?

Chapter 16
MISCELLANEOUS CALCULATIONS

In this chapter:
- *Insulin Measurement*
- *Temperature Conversion*
- *Automatic Compounders*

INSULIN MEASUREMENT

Insulin, a hormone necessary for regulation of blood sugar levels, is measured in units of activity. There are many types of insulin available including Regular, Semilente, NPH, Lente, PZI, Ultralente, and mixed NPH/Regular.

Note: *The only type of insulin which may be given IV is Regular!*

Points to Remember

- Regular insulin is available in concentrations of 40 units/ml (U/ml) and 100 u/ml. The labeling on insulin vials will state either U-100 (100 U/ml) or U-40 (40 U/ml). U-100 insulin is by far the most commonly used in practice.

- There are specialized insulin syringes available which measure the insulin in units directly. However, these syringes may not always be available, so it is important to know how to measure insulin by volume.

- Measuring insulin is similar to measuring any other liquid having a known concentration.

Examples

1. *Measure out 40 units of U-100 insulin:*

$$40 \text{ units} \times \frac{1 \text{ ml}}{100 \text{ units}} = \frac{40 \text{ ml}}{100} \text{ or } 0.4 \text{ ml}$$

2. Measure out 40 units of U-40 insulin:

$$40 \text{ units} \times \frac{1 \text{ ml}}{40 \text{ units}} = 1 \text{ ml}$$

❖ PRACTICE PROBLEMS

1. Given U-100 insulin, give the appropriate volume for the following:
   1. 10 units
   2. 20 units
   3. 30 units
   4. 60 units
   5. 80 units
   6. 90 units

2. Given U-40 insulin, give the appropriate volume for the following:
   7. 80 units
   8. 60 units
   9. 40 units
   10. 36 units
   11. 32 units
   12. 16 units
   13. 20 units
   14. 12 units
   15. 8 units

TEMPERATURE CONVERSION

In the United States, temperature is most commonly measured using the Fahrenheit scale. However, as is so often the case, the rest of the world uses another standard: the Celsius or centigrade scale.

Points to Remember
- The Centigrade scale was established for ease of use similar to that of the metric system. On this scale, water at sea level will boil at 100° and freeze at 0°.
- This is in contrast to the Fahrenheit scale, which measures the boiling point of water at 212° and establishes the freezing point of water as 32°.

Sometimes a temperature measured by one scale will need to be converted to the other. Two formulas are used to accomplish this:

a. $$\text{degrees Fahrenheit} = (\text{degrees celsius} + 40) \times \frac{9}{5} - 40$$

b. $$\text{degrees Celsius} = (\text{Fahrenheit} + 40) \times \frac{5}{9} - 40$$

122 *Miscellaneous Calculations*

👉 CHECK YOUR UNDERSTANDING

1. Convert 98.6° Fahrenheit to degrees Celsius:
Solution:

$$\text{degrees Celsius} = (\text{Fahrenheit} + 40) \times \frac{5}{9} - 40$$

degrees Celsius = $(98.6 + 40) \times \frac{5}{9} - 40$

Answer: degrees Celsius = 37

2. Convert 40° Celsius to Fahrenheit:
Solution:

$$\text{degrees Fahrenheit} = (\text{degrees Celsius} + 40) \times \frac{9}{5} - 40$$

degrees Fahrenheit = $(40 + 40) \times \frac{9}{5} - 40$

Answer: degrees Fahrenheit = 104

❖ PRACTICE PROBLEMS

Convert the following to degrees Celsius. (Round to one decimal place.)

1. 0° F	2. 10° F	3. 20° F	4. 32° F
5. 50° F	6. 72° F	7. 90° F	8. 110°F
9. 150° F	10. 165° F	11. 212° F	12. 300° F

Convert the following to degrees Fahrenheit. (Round to 1 decimal place.)

13. -41° C	14. -20°C	15. -5° C	16. 0° C
17. 10° C	18. 25° C	19. 38° C	20. 41° C
21. 45° C	22. 105° C		

AUTOMATIC COMPOUNDERS

In many hospitals and home health care facilities, the volume of custom-made intravenous mixtures is very high. In most of these instances, both space and skilled help are at a premium, so these facilities have turned to automation. A variety of machines have been developed which can pump components of intravenous admixtures from bulk containers into a final container which may be administered to the patient. Those compounders can move fluid many times faster than can a human using a syringe.

These compounders are wonderful, but they still require some human input to do their job; therefore, a knowledge of the principles upon which they work is necessary. There are numerous different automatic compounder designs on the market. Some rely on very simple principles, and others utilize a more complex interaction between the bulk containers and the final container.

Points to Remember
The various principles utilized are listed below:
- **Volume:** The simplest compounders are merely pumps that utilize flexible tubing made especially for that compounder and a rotating cam pressed against it which squeezes the liquid out of the short section of that tubing into the final bag. After the machine is calibrated for a specific solution type (such as NS or D$_5$W) and a specific needle size, a microprocessor remembers how many revolutions of the cam it will take to deliver any volume.
- **Weight:** The more complicated compounders weigh the bulk bottle, the final bag, or both. When the user inputs the **specific gravity** and desired **volume** of a solution into the compounder, a microprocessor determines how much that amount of fluid should weigh. The compounder will then pump the solution into the final bag (using the same setup as volume compounders) until this weight is achieved.
- The latter type of compounder is more accurate than the former because it cannot be thrown off calibration if the tubing stretches out of shape or if the tubing is of irregular size.

SPECIFIC GRAVITY

Specific gravity is a measure of weight of a given volume of a substance relative to the same volume of a standard when both have the same temperature. For solids and liquids, the standard is water. To determine specific gravity:

specific gravity = weight of substance ÷ weight of an equal volume of water

---

📖 CHECK YOUR UNDERSTANDING

1. 100 milliliters of 50% dextrose in water solution weighs 117 grams: if 100 ml of water weighs 100 grams, what is the specific gravity of D$_{50}$?

Solution:

Specific gravity of D$_{50}$ = 117 grams ÷ 100 grams

Answer: Specific gravity of D$_{50}$ = 1.17

The preceding example shows that D$_{50}$ weighs 1.17 times more than an equal volume of water, no matter what the volume.

This formula is used infrequently as specific gravities for most substances to be compounded will be provided.

A More Useful Formula:

weight of final volume (grams) = volume desired (ml) × specific gravity

The final weight is measured in grams because 1 ml of water weighs one gram and specific gravity is measured in relation to water. Therefore, the specific gravity of a substance is actually how much 1 ml of that substance weighs.

The above formula is useful for double-checking the accuracy of the compounder. This is done by comparing the actual weight of the solution created with the weight predicted by the equation; if the two do not match, or are not within the tolerance limits established by the institution (usually ± 5-10%), then the compounder is not accurate and must be recalibrated.

✍ CHECK YOUR UNDERSTANDING

If 500 ml of D$_{70}$ (specific gravity = 1.24) are to be transferred to a container from a bulk bottle, how much should the solution weigh?

Solution:

weight of solution = 500 × 1.24

Answer: weight of solution = 620 grams

❖ PRACTICE PROBLEMS

Given 100 ml of water = 100 grams:

1. If 100 ml of a substance weighs 88 grams, what is its specific gravity?
2. What would the specific gravity of a substance be if 100 ml weighed 200 grams?
3. The specific gravity of a substance is 1.17. How much would 250 ml weigh?
4. How much would 500 ml of a substance having a specific gravity of 0.9 weigh?
5. If 50 ml of a substance weighs 55 grams, what is its specific gravity?
   (**Hint:** Remember that specific gravity is a relationship between **equal** volumes of water and the substance)
6. If 500 ml of substance A (specific gravity = 1.1) and 250 ml of substance B (specific gravity = 1.25) are added to the same bag, what will the bag weigh?
7. An automatic compounder is programmed to measure 200 ml of D$_{50}$ (specific gravity = 1.17). If the final weight of the solution is found to be 250 grams, has the compound delivered the solution accurately?

For the following questions, give the weight of the solution:

8. 1,000 ml of D$_{50}$ (specific gravity = 1.12)
9. 900 ml of D$_{70}$ (specific gravity = 1.24)
10. 750 ml of a solution having a specific gravity of 1.01
11. 200 ml of a solution have a specific gravity of 1.1

Given the weight and volume of a solution, calculate its specific gravity:

	Volume	Weight
12.	100 ml	120 grams
13.	500 ml	1 kilogram
14.	750 ml	750 grams
15.	900 ml	990 grams
16.	1 liter	4 kilograms

Chapter 17
DILUTIONS

In this chapter:
- *Understanding Dilutions*
- *Preparing Dilutions*

UNDERSTANDING DILUTIONS

Many times in practice, pharmacy personnel are confronted with doses that are much too small to be measured accurately given the concentrations supplied by the manufacturer. These situations are most often encountered when:

- *Drugs are being dosed for neonatal use.*

- *A patient is allergic to a drug that is urgently needed. Very small doses of that drug may be given to desensitize the patient—a way to temporarily "short-circuit" the allergic response.*

- *Amounts of solid drug products are so small that they can not be directly measured because the scale being used is not sensitive enough.*

When these situations occur, a common response is to add a relatively inert ingredient in a sufficient quantity to dilute the original concentration down so that it may be accurately measured. The resulting product is sometimes referred to as an **aliquot**.

Points to Remember

Steps involved in creation of dilutions:
- Determine a final concentration that will allow the dose to be measured accurately. This figure may be chosen arbitrarily; however, final concentrations in base ten are the easiest to measure (i.e. $10mg/ml$ $100g/L$ $1000g/L$).

126 Dilutions

- Determine an amount of the manufacturer's drug product that can be measured easily. (This value may also be chosen arbitrarily, but the total amount of drug needed should be kept in mind so as to create enough dilution to complete the task but not so much as to create a lot of waste.)
- 2 ÷ 1 = final amount of diluted substance to be created.
- 3 − 2 = approximate amount of diluent to create the final product. (The value is approximate because the physical properties of some chemicals cause small amounts of volume contraction or expansion.)

CHECK YOUR UNDERSTANDING

1. Gentamicin is supplied to your pharmacy as a 40 mg/ml solution. Create a dilution that will allow the measurement of a 1 mg dose.

Solution:

a. Final concentration needed = 10 mg/ml (a 1 mg dose would be 0.1 ml)

b. Amount of drug that may be measured accurately = 40 mg

c. $40 \text{ mg} \div \frac{10 \text{ mg}}{\text{ml}} \rightarrow \text{rearrange} \rightarrow 40 \text{ mg} \times \frac{\text{ml}}{10 \text{ mg}} = 4 \text{ ml}$

Final amount of diluted product = 4 ml

d. 4 ml − 1 ml (40 mg) = 3 ml diluent (approx)

Answer: 3 ml diluent, 1 ml concentrated stock solution.

Hint: Before proficiency is attained, it is easiest to choose an amount that is equal to 1 ml for liquid dose forms and values such as 1, 10, 100 etc. for solid quantities. This technique will make calculations easier by eliminating mental clutter.

2. Dilute a 4 mg/ml solution so that 0.2 mg doses may be measured accurately.

Solution:

a. Final concentration desired = 1 mg/ml (a 0.2 mg dose would then be 0.2 ml)

b. Amount of initial product to be measured = 4 mg (1 ml)

c. Final amount of diluted product:

$$4 \text{ mg} \div \frac{1 \text{ mg}}{\text{ml}} \rightarrow 4 \text{ mg} \times \frac{\text{ml}}{1 \text{ mg}} = 4 \text{ ml}$$

d. Approximate amount of diluent required:

$$4 \text{ ml} - 1 \text{ ml } (40 \text{ mg}/1\text{m}) = 3 \text{ ml}$$

Answer: 3 ml

Note: In step #4, one would actually add a sufficient quantity to make the volume found in #3; most often this will be the answer found in #4, but sometimes it will be a little less or a little more.

3. A 0.02 mg dose of atropine is required for a child. However, the balance that you have cannot directly measure this quantity. Dilute the atropine with lactose to a concentration that will allow the 0.02 mg to be contained in 1 mg of the atropine/lactose mixture.

Solution:

a. Final concentration desired:

$$\frac{0.02 \text{ mg atropine}}{1 \text{ mg mixture}}$$

b. Amount of atropine to be measured:

$$1 \text{ mg (arbitrarily chosen)}$$

c. Total amount of atropine/lactose to be created:

$$1 \text{ mg atropine} \times \frac{1 \text{ mg mixture}}{0.02 \text{ mg atropine}} = 50 \text{ mg mixture}$$

d. Approximate amount of lactose needed:

$$50 \text{ mg} - 1 \text{ mg} = 49 \text{ mg lactose}$$

Answer: 49 mg lactose, 1 mg atropine

4. *You are instructed to make ten doses of a dilution of cefazolin. Each dose is to be 7.5 mg. The initial concentration of cefazolin is 100 mg/ml. Create a dilution that will be enough to manufacture these doses with only a small amount of wastage.*

Solution:

a. Final concentration desired = 10 mg/ml

b. Amount of cefazolin to be measured:

$$7.5 \text{ mg (size of each dose)} \times 10 \text{ (\# of doses needed)} = 75 \text{ mg}$$

Round up to a quantity more easily measured

Answer: 80 mg

c. $80 \text{ mg} \times \frac{\text{ml}}{10 \text{ mg}} = 8 \text{ ml dilution}$

d. $8 \text{ ml} - 0.8 \text{ ml} (80 \text{ mg}) = 7.2 \text{ ml diluent needed}$

$$7.5 \text{ mg} \div \frac{10 \text{ mg}}{\text{ml}} \rightarrow 7.5 \text{ mg} \times \frac{\text{ml}}{10 \text{ mg}} = 0.75 \text{ ml}$$

Answer: Each dose would be 0.75 ml, using 7.2 ml diluent and 0.8 ml concentrated stock solution.

❖ PRACTICE PROBLEMS

Answer the problems below using the following initial concentrations:

Gentamicin—20 mg/ml

Dexamethasone—4 mg/ml

Digoxin—50 mcg/ml

Nafcillin—250 mg/ml

Metoclopramide—5 mg/ml

Morphine—10 mg/ml

Ondansetron—2 mg/ml

Penicillin—500,000 U/ml

1. Make a dilution of ondansetron that will allow a dose of 0.001 mg to be measured easily.
2. 25 doses of gentamicin 8 mg must be prepared. Create a 10 mg/ml dilution of appropriate volume that will satisfy this requirement. (You may round the volume up to make the calculation easier.)
3. Prepare a 5 mcg/ml dilution of digoxin having a final volume of 5 ml.

4. 10 ml of a 0.5 mg/ml dilution of metoclopramide is desired. What volume of metoclopramide stock is required?
5. 5 doses of morphine 0.8 mg are desired. Prepare enough of a 1 mg/ml dilution to dispense all the doses needed.
6. Prepare 20 ml of a 25 mg/ml nafcillin dilution.
7. Prepare 10 ml of a 1 mg/ml dexamethasone dilution.
8. A dose of 0.6 mg gentamicin is needed for a patient. Three of these doses are to be prepared at a time. Prepare a dilution of sufficient concentration and volume to prepare these doses.
9. 20 nafcillin 12.5 mg doses are to be prepared. Make a 25 mg/ml dilution that will satisfy this requirement.
10. Prepare a dexamethasone dilution from which one may dispense the following doses:
    a. 5 × 0.4 mg doses
    b. 3 × 0.6 mg doses
    c. 8 × 0.2 mg doses
    d. 12 × 0.1 mg doses

11. Prepare the following penicillin dilutions with the knowledge that 0.1 ml will be used from each dilution.
    a. 100 U/ml   b. 250 U/ml
    c. 500 U/ml   d. 1500 U/ml
    e. 10,000 U/ml   f. 50,000 U/ml
    g. 150,000 U/ml   h. 250,000 U/ml

12. Prepare a 10 mcg/ml solution of digoxin having a final volume of 3 ml. How many ml of digoxin 50 mcg/ml will be needed?

Chapter 18
ELECTROLYTE CALCULATIONS

In this chapter:
- *The Milliequivalent*
- *Successful Conversions*
- *Calculating Meq for Compounds*
- *Preparation of Saline Solutions*

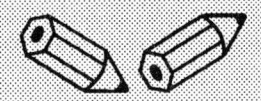

DEFINING ELECTROLYTES

Many liquids are used in pharmacy practice which contain salts in solution. These salts are also referred to as **electrolytes** *because, when dissolved in water, they will conduct electricity.*

When the electrolyte in question is sodium chloride, the solution may also be called a saline solution. When any other electrolyte is being used, the common or chemical name of the salt will be used, i.e., magnesium sulfate solution or $MgSo_4$ solution.

Points to Remember

- Almost all solutions have their electrolytes measured by the milliequivalent (mEq). The meaning of the mEq will be explained later.
- The creation of solutions for patient use is achieved by adding a measured quantity of a more concentrated electrolyte solution to an ordered diluting solution (stock solution).
- The content of these concentrated electrolyte solutions is measured almost exclusively in milliequivalents/ml (mEq/ml).

To determine what volume of concentrated electrolyte solution to use in preparation, use the following formula.

$$\text{ml concentrated solution needed} = \text{mEq needed} \times \frac{\text{ml}}{\text{mEq}}$$

130 Electrolyte Calculations

Example

A concentrated calcium gluconate (Cagluc) solution contains 0.465 mEq/ml. If 4.65 mEq of Cagluc are needed to prepare a solution, how many ml of this concentrated solution needs to be measured?

$$\text{ml needed} = 4.65 \times \frac{\text{ml}}{0.465} = 10\text{ml}$$

Alternative Method: Divide the quantity desired by the concentration:

$$4.65 \div 0.465 = 10\text{ml}$$

As may be recalled from a previous chapter, the methods used for finding volumes of electrolyte concentrates are the same as those employed in finding volumes of liquid drugs that are measured in mg/ml.

THE MILLIEQUIVALENT

Most electrolytes in pharmacy practice are measured by the milliequivalent. There are some exceptions to this statement and will be discussed later.

The equivalent (and subsequently, the milliequivalent) is a measure of an element's or ion's chemical combining power. The equivalent is measured in relation to hydrogen in that it measures the weight of ion or element that is required to achieve the same reactivity as 1 gram of hydrogen. The **valence** of an element or ion determines how many atoms or ions are required to form a stable compound with another element or ion. See the table of the elements, their valences and atomic weights located on page 131.

Consider: Hydrogen has a valence of 1, and oxygen has a valence of 2. Therefore, it takes two hydrogen atoms to form a stable compound with 1 oxygen atom (H_2O).

The equivalent takes both atomic weight and valence into account. To use the formula, remember that atomic weight is measured in grams.

FORMULA #1

$$1 \text{ equivalent weight} = \frac{\text{atomic weight}}{\text{valence}}$$

Example

Oxygen has an atomic weight of 16 and a valence of 2. What is the equivalent weight?

$$1 \text{ equivalent wt} = \frac{\text{atomic weight}}{\text{valence}}$$

$$\frac{16}{2} = 8$$

Therefore, 8 grams of oxygen have the same chemical reactivity as 1 gram of hydrogen.

Note: Valence is the important consideration in this formula, not whether that valence is negative or positive.

The milliequivalent (mEq) is merely the equivalent weight of the substance divided by 1000 (milli = one-thousandth).

Common Elements, Their Valences and Atomic Weights

Element	Symbol	Valence	Atomic Weight
Hydrogen	H	1	1.008
Helium	He	0	4.003
Lithium	Li	1	6.939
Carbon	C	2,4	12.011
Nitrogen	N	3,5	14.007
Oxygen	O	2	15.999
Flourine	F	1	18.998
Neon	Ne	0	20.179
Sodium	Na	1	22.9898
Magnesium	Mg	2	24.305
Aluminum	Al	3	26.982
Silicon	Si	4	28.086
Phosphorus	P	3,5	30.9738
Sulphur	S	2,4,6	32.064
Chlorine	Cl	1,3,5,7	35.453
Argon	Ar	0	39.948
Potassium	K	1	39.102
Calcium	Ca	2	40.08
Iron	Fe	2,3,4,6	55.847
Copper	Cu	1,2	63.546
Silver	Ag	1,2	107.868
Iodine	I	1,2,5,7	126.9044
Gold	Au	1,3	196.967
Mercury	Hg	1,2	200.59
Lead	Pb	2,4	207.19

132 Electrolyte Calculations

✎ CHECK YOUR UNDERSTANDING

1. Carbon has an atomic weight of 12 and a valence of 4. How much does one milliequivalent weigh?

a. $\quad 1 \text{ equivalent} = \dfrac{12 \text{ grams}}{4} = 3 \text{ grams}$

b. $\quad \dfrac{3 \text{ grams}}{1000} = 0.003 \text{ grams or 3 milligrams}$

At this point, the student is asked to look for a similarity in the preceding steps to solution, as this similarity is the key to the following shortcut formula:

$$1 \text{ milliequivalent} = \dfrac{\text{atomic wt}}{\text{valence}}$$

In this shortcut formula, the only change is in the **name** of the units of atomic weight—*grams* becomes *milligrams*. The numerical expression of atomic weight is **not** converted.

2. Carbon has an atomic weight of 12 and a valence of 4. How much does one milliequivalent weigh?

Using the Shortcut Formula

$$1 \text{ milliequivalent} = \dfrac{12 \text{ milligrams}}{4} = 3 \text{ milligrams}$$

The shortcut automatically converts equivalent weight to milliequivalent weight because of this unit change.

If this shortcut is unclear, **do not use it** until it is understood. Remember, shortcuts are presented to make calculations easier; they should not be used if the student does not feel comfortable with them.

CONVERSIONS

A substance may be converted from mg to mEq and vice-versa by employing the following formula:

$$\# \text{ of mEqs present} = \dfrac{\text{weight of substance}}{\text{milliequivalent weight}}$$

To use this formula, one must first determine the mEq weight.

✎ CHECK YOUR UNDERSTANDING

1. Sodium has an atomic weight of 23 and a valence of 1. How many mEq are present in 46 mg of sodium?

Solution:

a. Find mEq weight using $1 \text{ mEq} = \dfrac{\text{atomic wt}}{\text{valence}} \div 1000$

or

$1 \text{ mEq} = \dfrac{\text{atomic wt}}{\text{valence}} \text{ mg (shortcut method)}$

$1 \text{ mEq} = \dfrac{23 \text{ g}}{1} \div 1000 = 23 \text{ mg}$

or

$$1 \text{ mEq} = \frac{23 \text{ mg}}{1} = 23 \text{ mg}$$

b. $\quad$ mEq present $= \dfrac{\text{mg present}}{\text{mEq wt}}$

$$\text{mEq present} = \frac{46 \text{ mg}}{23 \text{ mg}} = 2$$

Answer: 2 mEq are present in 46 mg of sodium

2. Find the weight of 4 mEq of calcium, given its atomic weight of 40 and valence of 2.

Solution:

a. $\quad$ Find mEq wt:

$$1 \text{ mEq} = \frac{40 \text{ g}}{2} \div 1000 = 20 \text{ mg} \quad \text{or} \quad 1 \text{ mEq} = \frac{40 \text{ mg}}{2} = 20 \text{ mg}$$

b. $\quad$ number of mEq present $= \dfrac{\text{wt of substance}}{\text{mEq wt}}$

$$4 \text{ mEq} = \frac{\text{weight of substance}}{20 \text{ mg}}$$
$$\downarrow$$
$$4 = \frac{x}{20} \rightarrow 4 \times 20 = x \rightarrow 80 = x$$

Answer: 4 mEq of calcium = 80 mg

CALCULATING MEQ FOR COMPOUNDS

Compounds can be measured in mEq in much the same manner as that which is used for single atoms.

The first step is to identify the empirical formula of the compound. Some examples of empirical formulas are: CO_2, H_2O, $CaCl_2$, NaCl, KCl, and $FeSO_4$. The next step is to fragment the empirical formula into its component atoms, i.e., $FeSO_4$ becomes Fe, S, O. Next, the atomic weight of each atom is multiplied by the quantity of those atoms in the compound. The values of this step are added together and placed into the mEq formula submitted earlier. The value for valence is determined by the atom or ion having the largest valence, i.e., H_2O—since oxygen has a valence of 2, this value will be used in the equation. Here, electrical charge **does** play a role in the calculation of mEq, not because of the charge itself but because of its resulting from the formation of ions.

For example, the ion SO_4 would not be broken down to individual sulfur and oxygen atoms to find which has the highest valence for use in calculating mEq. The valence of the ion will be used instead because the ion is what would react with hydrogen in a test for equivalency.

Example

Given H_2SO_4, with a molecular weight of 98, and valences of 1 for hydrogen and 2 for SO_4, determine how many mg one mEq weighs.

Solution:

a. $\quad 1 \text{ mEq} = \dfrac{98}{2} = 49$

$\quad$ **or**

b. 1 mEq = 49 mg H₂SO₄

The preceding formulas all depend on the substance in question possessing a measurable valence. However, not all substances have this quality. The most notable examples are the so-called "noble" gases: helium, xenon, krypton, neon and argon. These gases possess no valence and will react with no other atom unless exposed to unnatural forces.

Another exception is the phosphate ion, which is commonly dealt with in the practice of pharmacy. This ion possesses the potential to change its valence and the quantity of oxygen it contains depending on pH and temperature. Several different ions containing phosphorus and oxygen often occupy the same solution and all are called "phosphate."

In a case such as that encountered with phosphate, the substance will be measured in moles or millimoles rather than in milliequivalents.

One mole is equivalent to the atomic weight of the substance, and one millimole (mM) is: one mole ÷ 1000. Since the atomic weight of a substance is measured in grams, so is the mole.

Example

Chlorine has an atomic weight of 35.5. How much does one millimole (mM) weigh?

$$1mM = \frac{35.5 \text{ grams}}{1000} = 0.0355 \text{ g or } 35.5 \text{ mg}$$

Shortcut

Here, a shortcut method similar to that used in the calculation of mEq may be employed. Since 1mm = 1 mole ÷ 1000 and 1 mg = 1 gram ÷ 1000, the numerical value of 1 mM is the same as for 1 mole. The only difference is the units employed.

SALINE PREPARATIONS

Saline preparations are solutions of sodium chloride. These solutions are measured relative to a standard which is referred as "normal saline" or "NS". Normal saline is a 0.9% sodium chloride solution. That is, 100 ml of solution contains 0.9 grams of sodium chloride.

Saline solutions having concentrations greater than or equal to 0.9% have a wide variety of names attached to them, some of which are not technically correct. Consider the following table:

Sodium Chloride Concentrations and Their Common Names

Actual Sodium Chloride Concentration	Common Names
0.9%	Normal Saline or NS
0.45%	one-half Normal Saline or ½ NS or 0.45 NS
0.225%	one-quarter NS or ¼ NS or 0.2 NS

As the chart shows, 0.225% sodium chloride is sometimes incorrectly referred to as "0.2 NS." Knowing this information prior to having to dispense this particular solution should eliminate some confusion.

PREPARATION OF VARIOUS SALINE SOLUTIONS

While IV solution manufacturers strive to create a wide variety of saline concentrations and volumes for use in intravenous preparations, it is not feasible for manufacturers to make all the possible concentrations, nor will a pharmacy stock all of those manufactured, for to do this would be akin to committing economic suicide. Therefore, unconventional saline concentrations will sometimes need to be prepared.

When the student has memorized the following equivalence, the remainder of this section will be relatively easy:

1 liter of normal saline contains 154 mEq of sodium chloride.

This statement is important because to make non-standard saline concentrations, one must use a concentrated sodium chloride solution. These solutions list their concentrations in mEq/ml; therefore, one must know how many mEq of sodium chloride are needed to prepare the desired saline solution.

To show why 154 mEq of sodium chloride/liter of NS is equivalent to 0.9% sodium chloride solution, the following is submitted:

a. 1 liter NS = 0.9% sodium chloride

b. $0.9\% = \dfrac{0.9 \text{ grams}}{100 \text{ ml}}$ **or** $\dfrac{9 \text{ grams}}{1000 \text{ ml}}$ **or** $\dfrac{9000 \text{ mg}}{1000 \text{ ml}}$

c. Sodium (Na) has an atomic wt of 23 and a valence of 1 Chlorine (Cl) has an atomic wt of 35.5 and a valence of 1

so

$1 \text{ mEq NaCl} = \dfrac{23 + 35.5}{1} = 58.5 \text{ mg}$ (**Remember:** Use only the largest valence.)

d. Recall the formula for converting mg to mEq:

$\text{mEq of substance in question} = \dfrac{\text{mg of substance}}{\text{milliequivalent wt}}$

so

$\text{mEq of substance} = \dfrac{9000}{58.5}$ **or** 153.846 **or** 154 mEq

e. Therefore: 0.9% sodium chloride solution contains 153.846 or 154 mEq of NaCl.

Armed with that equivalency, it is relatively easy to know exactly how many mEq of NaCl must be added to sterile water to create a desired volume of saline solution.

The easiest method to show on paper is the following formula:

$\text{mEq NaCl needed} = \dfrac{154 \text{ mEq}}{\text{liter of NS}} \times \text{volume desired (liter)} \times \text{fraction of NS desired}$

Where:

Volume desired is expressed in whole or partial liters and fraction of NS desired refers to such values as ¼ NS, ½ NS, and ¾ NS. This formula uses the NaCl content of 1 liter of NS as its base:

$$\dfrac{154 \text{ mEq}}{(1 \text{ liter of NS})}$$

From there, it reduces or enlarges 154 mEq according to the volume to be prepared (volume desired). Lastly, a conversion is made from a desired volume expressed as NS to a volume expressed as the desired fraction of NS.

✍ CHECK YOUR UNDERSTANDING

1. How many mEq of NaCl are required to make 1 liter of NS?
Solution:

$$\text{mEq NaCl required} = \frac{154 \text{ mEq}}{1 \text{ L NS}} \times 1\text{L} \times 1(\text{NS}) = 154 \text{ mEq are required}$$

2. Find the amount of NaCl required to make 500 ml (½ liter) of ½ NS.

$$\text{mEq required} = \frac{154 \text{ mEq}}{1 \text{L NS}} \times \frac{1}{2}\text{L} \times \frac{1}{2}\text{NS} = \frac{154}{4} \text{ or } 38.5 \text{ mEq}$$

3. How many mEq of NaCl are required to prepare 250 ml (¼ liter) of ¾ NS?

$$\text{mEq NaCl required} = \frac{154 \text{ mEq}}{1 \text{ L NS}} \times \frac{1}{4}\text{L} \times \frac{3}{4}\text{NS} = \frac{462}{16} \text{ or } 28.87 \text{ mEq}$$

Since syringes and other measuring devices can not measure milliequivalents, one must convert the answers found in the previous equations to milliliters of sodium chloride concentrate. Most commercially available concentrated sodium chloride solutions contain 4 mEq NaCl/ml. Knowing this, one may proceed in two ways:

1. Convert mEq to ml in a second step;
2. Add the 4 mEq/ml conversion factor to formula 1.

The following example will be solved using both methods.

✍ CHECK YOUR UNDERSTANDING

1. How many ml of a 4 mEq/ml NaCl solution are needed to prepare 500 ml of ¼ NS?
Solution # 1:

a. $\quad \text{mEq required} = \dfrac{154 \text{ mEq}}{\text{liter NS}} \times \dfrac{1}{2} \text{ liter} \times \dfrac{1}{4}\text{NS} = \dfrac{154}{8} = 19.25 \text{ mEq}$

b. $\quad \text{ml desired} = 19.25 \text{ mEq} \times \dfrac{1 \text{ ml}}{4 \text{ mEq}} = \dfrac{19.25}{4} \text{ or } 4.81 \text{ ml}$

Answer: 4.81 ml of sodium chloride concentrate are needed.

Solution # 2: (add 4 mEq/ml conversion factor)

$$\text{ml required} = \frac{154 \text{ mEq}}{\text{liter NS}} \times \frac{1}{2} \text{ liter} \times \frac{1}{4} \text{NS} \times \frac{1 \text{ ml}}{4 \text{ mEq}} = \frac{154}{32} \text{ or } 4.81 \text{ ml}$$

Once one has found the volume of sodium chloride concentrate to be used in the preparation of a saline solution, this volume must be subtracted from the total volume, giving the volume of sterile water to be used. Of course, if other liquids are to be added, their volumes must also be subtracted.

2. Prepare 1 liter of ¼ NS which also contains 10 ml of potassium chloride (KCl) concentrate.
Solution:

a. $\quad \text{ml NaCl concentrate} = \dfrac{154 \text{mEq}}{1 \text{ liter NS}} \times 1 \text{ liter} \times \dfrac{1}{4}\text{NS} \times \dfrac{1 \text{ml}}{4 \text{mEq}} = \dfrac{154}{16}$

   or 9.6 ml

b. $\quad 1000\text{ml} - 9.6 \text{ ml} - 10\text{ml} = 980.4\text{ml}$

So, to make 1000 ml of ¼ NS with 10 ml KCl solution, one must have 980.4 ml sterile water, 10 ml KCl concentrate, and 9.6 ml NaCl concentrate.

❖ PRACTICE PROBLEMS

1. Magnesium sulfate (MgSO$_4$) solution contains 4 mEq/ml as MgSO$_4$. If 12 meq are needed, how many ml are needed?
2. If a solution of potassium chloride (KCl) contains 2 mEq/ml, how many mEq are contained in 10 ml?
3. Calcium has an atomic weight of 40 and a valence of 2. How much does 16 mEq weigh?
4. If iron has an atomic weight of 55.85, how much does 1 millimole weigh?

Create the following solutions (round all answers to one decimal place). (For the following questions, sterile water, and sodium chloride (NaCl) 4 mEq/ml will be used.)

5. 250 ml (¼ L) of ½ NS
6. 2 Liters of ¾ NS
7. 750 ml of ½ NS
8. 500 ml of ⅓ NS
9. 300 ml of ½ NS
10. 400 ml of ¼ NS
11. Hydrogen chloride has an atomic weight of 36.5. If hydrogen and chlorine both have valences of 1, how much does 1 mEq weigh?
12. *Given the following information:*

    Atomic weight of Mg = 24.31

    valence of Mg = 2

    Atomic weight of SO$_4$ = 96

    valence of SO$_4$ = 2

    How many mEq are contained in 1.804 grams MgSO$_4$? (round to one decimal place)

13. How much does 15 mEq of CaCl$_2$ weigh?
14. What is the weight of 10 millimoles of MgSO$_4$?
15. Calcium gluconate is supplied in a concentration of 0.465 mEq/ml. How many ml are required to supply a 9.3 mEq dose?

Chapter 19
PERCENTAGE PREPARATIONS

In this chapter:
- *Percent Strength*
- *Specific and Non-specific Concentration Dosing*
- *Alligation Method of Calculation*
- *Dextrose in Saline Solutions*

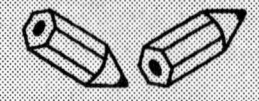

PERCENT STRENGTH

Percent strength is a method of quantifying a mixture's concentration. Rather than stating that a solution contains 1 gram of drug in 100 milliliters of solution, one would say that it is a 1% solution. Percent strength measures the quantity of a specified substance in 100 units of a specified mixture.

Points to Remember

There are three types of percent strength:

- w/w (weight/weight) measures grams of substance in 100 grams of mixture
- w/v (weight/volume) measures grams of substance in 100 milliliters of mixture
- v/v (volume/volume) measures milliliters of substance in 100 milliliters of mixture
- The most common measurement of this group is w/v; the other two are used only rarely.
- If a mixture is v/v or w/w there will normally be a v/v or w/w denotation after the percentage strength, i.e. 1% v/v or 2% w/w.
- If the substance is w/v, this denotation will not always be present. Also, if the substance is a solid, the w/w designation will be left off as there is no doubt as to how the substance will be measured.

Examples

w/v 5% dextrose in water = 5 g dextrose in each 100 ml of dextrose/water solution
v/v 20% orange oil in water = 20 ml of orange oil in each 100 ml of orange oil/water mixture
w/w 1% codeine in lactose = 1 gram of codeine in each 100 g of codeine/lactose mixture

PRACTICAL APPLICATIONS

There are two primary applications of the concept of percent strength: the deliverance of a specific size dose (i.e. 12.5 grams) or the creation of a non-standard concentration (i.e. 7.25%).

Specific Concentration Dosing

To deliver a requested dose given a specific concentration:

$$\frac{\text{Dose needed}}{\text{quantity of mixture needed}} = \frac{\text{Percent strength}}{100}$$

Note: This formula works for w/v, w/w, and v/v problems. One must only remember to place the correct units in their proper place.

For w/v:

$$\frac{\text{grams desired}}{x \text{ ml solution}} = \frac{\text{grams}}{100 \text{ ml}} \; (concentration)$$

For v/v:

$$\frac{\text{ml desired}}{x \text{ ml solution}} = \frac{\text{ml}}{100 \text{ ml}}$$

For w/w:

$$\frac{\text{grams desired}}{x \text{ grams mixture}} = \frac{\text{grams}}{100 \text{ grams}} \; (concentration)$$

✍ CHECK YOUR UNDERSTANDING

1. How many ml of a 25% w/v solution of mannitol are needed to deliver a 12.5 gram dose?

Solution:

a. $\dfrac{12.5 \text{ grams}}{x \text{ ml}} = \dfrac{25 \text{ grams}}{100 \text{ ml}}$

b. 1250 = 25x
   50 ml = x

Answer: 50 ml of mannitol 25% are needed

2. How many grams of a 0.5% w/w codeine/lactose mixture are needed to deliver 0.01 grams of codeine?

Solution:

a. $\dfrac{0.01 \text{ grams}}{x \text{ grams}} = \dfrac{0.5 \text{ grams}}{100 \text{ grams}}$

b. 1 = 0.5x

2 = x

Answer: 2 grams of codeine/lactose mixture are required

As may already be noted, the solutions to these examples are attained by using simple ratios and then testing for equivalency by cross-multiplication.

Shortcut

Rather than using the ratio/proportion method, a shortcut may be employed that utilizes the conversion of concentration to decimal form.

As may be recalled from the chapter on fractions and decimals, a fraction (such as $25/100$) may be converted to a decimal by dividing the numerator by the denominator. This concept is used to convert concentration to a decimal. This will yield the following:

Amount of mixture desired = ml or grams desired ÷ concentration (expressed as a decimal)

Note: Units for ml or g desired depends on whether problem is w/v or v/v or w/w.

✍ CHECK YOUR UNDERSTANDING

1. How many ml of a 25% w/v mannitol solution are required to provide a 12.5 gram dose?

Solution:

a. $\quad$ ml of 25% solution = 12.5 g ÷ $\frac{0.25 \text{ g}}{\text{ml}}$ (25%)

b. $\quad$ ml of 25% solution = 12.5 g × $\frac{\text{ml}}{0.25 \text{ g}}$ → $\frac{12.5 \text{ ml}}{0.25}$ → 50 ml

Answer: 50 ml

Non-Standard Concentration Dosing

The second application of percent strength is the creation of non-standard solutions. As with saline concentrations, it is not feasible for a manufacturer or pharmacy to carry all possible concentrations of drugs. If a required concentration of a drug is not carried, it may be manufactured by diluting a more concentrated stock solution of that drug. For example, a 15% dextrose in water solution may be created by using 50% dextrose solution and sterile water. To create these non-standard solutions, the following formula may be employed:

ml of stock solution = {total volume needed (ml) × final concentration} ÷ concentration of stock solution

Where: stock solution = solution of drug supplied by the manufacturer

and:

Concentrations are expressed as a decimal or as $\frac{\text{Grams}}{100 \text{ ml}}$

This is how the formula works:

1. Total volume needed (ml) × **final concentration**—this portion of the formula establishes the gram quantity of the drug needed

2. This portion takes the gram quantity found in the first portion and converts it to milliliters of stock solution

CHECK YOUR UNDERSTANDING

1. How many ml of 50% dextrose (D_{50}) are required to create 200 ml of 10% dextrose (D_{10})?

Solution:

a. $\{200 \text{ ml} \times \dfrac{0.1 \text{ g}}{\text{ml}}\} \div \dfrac{0.5 \text{ g}}{\text{ml}}$

b. $20 \text{ g} \div \dfrac{0.5 \text{ g}}{\text{ml}} \rightarrow 20 \text{ g} \times \dfrac{\text{ml}}{0.5 \text{ g}} = 10 \text{ ml}$

Remember: Dividing by a fraction is the same as multiplying by the reciprocal of that fraction

Answer = 10 ml of D_{50}

2. How many ml of D_{70} are required to create 1 Liter of D_{15}?

Solution:

a. $\{1000 \text{ ml} \times \dfrac{0.15 \text{ g}}{\text{ml}}\} \div \dfrac{0.7 \text{ g}}{\text{ml}}$

b. $150 \text{ g} \div \dfrac{0.7 \text{ g}}{\text{ml}} \rightarrow 150 \text{ g} \times \dfrac{\text{ml}}{0.7 \text{ g}} = 214.2 \text{ ml}$

Answer: 214.2 ml of D_{70}

Of course, it takes more than just concentrated dextrose stock solution to create a dextrose in water IV. Sterile water must also be used in such a volume that it **plus** the stock dextrose will equal the final volume needed. This yields the following:

volume of sterile water needed = total volume needed − volume of dextrose stock solution

Example

From the first example: 10 ml of D_{50} were needed to make 200 ml of D_{10}. How many ml of sterile water are needed?

Solution:

200 ml solution − 10 ml D_{50} = 190 ml sterile water

As was mentioned earlier, percentage preparations in pharmacy are mostly calculations involving dextrose. However, many other substances can be measured by percentage strength.

CHECK YOUR UNDERSTANDING

1. *Using normal saline (NS) and bupivacaine 0.5%, create a 100 ml 0.125% bupivacaine in NS solution.*

Solution:

a. $\dfrac{0.125 \text{ g}}{100} \times 100 \text{ ml} \div \dfrac{0.5 \text{ g}}{100 \text{ ml}}$

b. Convert $\div \dfrac{0.5 \text{ g}}{100 \text{ m}}$ to $\times \dfrac{100 \text{ ml}}{0.5 \text{ g}}$ and cancel all units

$0.125 \times \dfrac{100 \text{ ml}}{0.5} = \dfrac{12.5 \text{ ml}}{0.5} \rightarrow 25 \text{ ml } 0.5\%$ bupivacaine

c. 100 ml solution − 25 ml bupivacaine = 75 ml saline

Answer: 25 ml bupivacaine and 75 ml NS

142 *Percentage Preparations*

ALLIGATION METHOD OF CALCULATION

Another useful tool in calculation of percentage preparations is alligation. This method uses a sort of graph resembling a tic-tac-toe board to find a solution. The graph has this appearance:

Most concentrated solution (B)		Parts of most concentrated solution needed (D)
	Final concentration desired (A)	
Least concentrated solution (C)		Parts of least concentrated solution needed (E)

Total parts of final concentration (F)

The formulas needed are as follows:

1. $B - A = E$
2. $A - C = D$
3. $D + E = F$

By comparing the graph with the formula, it becomes apparent that this method is not complicated.

Note: The most concentrated solution of the substance in question **always** appears on the upper left of the graph.

✍ CHECK YOUR UNDERSTANDING

1. Using D_{70} (70% dextrose solution) and water, how many parts of D_{70} and water are needed to create D_{30} (30% dextrose solution)?

70		
	30	
0 (water is 0% dextrose)		

→

70		30 parts of D_{70}
	30	
0		40 parts of water

70 total parts

Answer: 30 parts of D_{70} and 40 parts of water are needed.

From this beginning, any volume of D_{30} may be created by using the following formulas:

$$\frac{30 \text{ parts } D_{70}}{70 \text{ parts } D_{30}} = \frac{x \text{ ml } D_{70}}{x \text{ ml } D_{30}} \text{ and } \frac{40 \text{ parts water}}{70 \text{ parts } D_{30}} = \frac{x \text{ ml water}}{x \text{ ml } D_{30}}$$

2. Create 200 ml D_{30} from the above examples. List the total volumes of D_{70} and water needed.
Solution:

$$\frac{30 \text{ parts } D_{70}}{70 \text{ parts } D_{30}} = \frac{x \text{ ml } D_{70}}{200 \text{ml } D_{30}} \rightarrow 30 \times 200 = 70x$$
$$6000 = 70x$$
$$85.71 = x$$

Answer: 85.71 ml of D_{70} are needed.

$$\frac{40 \text{ parts water}}{70 \text{ parts } D_{30}} = \frac{x \text{ ml water}}{200 \text{ ml } D_{30}} \rightarrow 40 \times 200 = 70x$$
$$8000 = 70x$$
$$114.29 = x$$

Answer: 114.29 ml of water are needed.

3. Using D_{70} and D_{50}, create 500 ml of D_{60}.
Solution:
a.

70			70			70		10 parts D_{70}
	60	$\rightarrow$		60	$\rightarrow$		60	
50			50	10		50		10 parts D_{50}

20 parts D_{60}

b. $\dfrac{10 \text{ parts } D_{70}}{20 \text{ parts } D_{60}} = \dfrac{x \text{ ml } D_{70}}{500 \text{ml } D_{60}} \rightarrow 20x = 5000 \rightarrow x = 250$

Answer: 250 ml D_{70} are required.

c. $\dfrac{10 \text{ parts } D_{50}}{20 \text{ parts } D_{60}} = \dfrac{x \text{ ml } D_{50}}{500 \text{ ml } D_{60}} \rightarrow 20x = 5000 \rightarrow x = 250$

Answer: 250 ml D_{50} are required.

Final Answer: 250 ml of D_{70} and 250 ml D_{50} are required to prepare 500 ml of D_{60}.

Alligation works for any percent preparation, not just for dextrose solutions.

144 *Percentage Preparations*

4. Create 100 ml of 0.0625% bupivacaine in NS using 0.5% bupivacaine:
Solution:
a.

0.5%		0.0625 parts 0.5% bupivacaine
	0.0625%	
NS 0%		0.4375 parts NS
		0.5

b. $\dfrac{0.625}{0.5} = \dfrac{x}{100}$
$6.25 = 0.5x$
$12.5 = x$

c. **Answer:** 12.5 ml 0.5% bupivacaine are required to make 100 ml 0.0625% bupivacaine in NS.

d. **Final answer:** 100 − 12.5 = 87.5 ml NS are required.

DEXTROSE IN SALINE CALCULATIONS

Many of the solutions used in the pharmacy are not solely composed of dextrose or saline but a combination of the two.

To create dextrose and saline solutions, one simply does the calculations involved in finding the amount of concentrated dextrose and sodium chloride solutions needed to create the solution. Then, these volumes are subtracted from the total volume of solution to be created. The resulting answer will be the amount of sterile water needed to prepare the solution.

✍ CHECK YOUR UNDERSTANDING

1. Create a 1000 ml (1 liter) solution of 7.5% dextrose and ¼ normal saline ($D_{7.5}$ ¼ NS) using D_{50}, sodium chloride 4 mEq/ml and sterile water:

Solution:

a. Find volume of D_{50} stock solution needed:

$$1000 \text{ ml} \times \dfrac{7.5 \text{ g}}{100 \text{ ml}} \div \dfrac{50 \text{ g}}{100 \text{ ml}} \rightarrow 1000 \text{ ml} \times \dfrac{7.5 \text{ g}}{100 \text{ ml}} \times \dfrac{100 \text{ ml}}{50 \text{ g}} = 150 \text{ ml}$$

Answer: 150 ml of D_{50} are needed.

b. Find the volume of NaCl 4 mEq/ml needed:

$$\dfrac{154 \text{ mEq}}{1 \text{ L NS}} \times 1 \text{ liter} \times \dfrac{1}{4}\text{NS} \times \dfrac{1 \text{ ml}}{4 \text{ mEq}} = 9.62 \text{ ml}$$

Answer: 9.62 ml NaCl concentrate are needed.

c. Subtract D_{50} and NaCl volumes to find sterile water:

$$1000 \text{ ml} - 150 \text{ ml} - 9.62 \text{ ml} = 740.38 \text{ ml sterile water}$$

Final Answer: 150 ml D_{50}, 9.62 ml NaCl, 840.38 ml sterile water to make 1 Liter of $D_{7.5}$ ¼ NS

2. Create 1 liter of $D_{12.5}$ ½NS using D_{70}, NaCl 4 mEq/ml and sterile water. (This example will use percent strength converted to decimal form in the dextrose portion of the calculations.)

Solution:

a. Find the ml of D_{70} required:

$$1000 ml \times 0.125 \div 0.7 = 178.57 ml \ D_{70}$$

b. Find the ml of NaCl 4 mEq/ml required:

$$\frac{154 \ mEq}{1 \ L \ NS} \times 1 \ L \times \frac{1}{2} NS \times \frac{1 \ ml}{4 \ mEq} = 19.25 \ ml \ NaCl \ concentrate$$

c. Subtract volumes of D_{70} and NaCl to find the volume of sterile water required.

$$1000 \ ml - 178.57 \ ml - 19.25 \ ml = 802.18$$

Answer: To create 1 L of $D_{12.5}$ ½ NS, one would need 178.57 ml D_{70}, 19.25 NaCl 4 mEq/ml
and 802.18 ml sterile water.

3. Create 200 ml of $D_{12.5}$% ¼ NS using D_{50}, water, and NaCl 4 mEq/ml.

a.

50		12.5 Parts D_{50}
	12.5	
(NS is 0% bupivacaine)		37.5 Parts water
	50 Parts $D_{12.5}$	

$\rightarrow \quad \dfrac{12.5 \text{ parts } D_{50}}{50 \text{ parts } D_{12.5}} = \dfrac{x \text{ ml } D_{50}}{200 \text{ ml } D_{12.5}}$

Answer: 50 ml D_{50} are needed.

b. $\dfrac{154 \ mEq}{1 \ L \ NS} \times \dfrac{1}{4} NS \times 0.2 \ L \times \dfrac{1 \ ml}{4 mEq} = \dfrac{30.8}{16} \rightarrow$ 1.925 ml or 1.93 ml

c. $200 - 50 - 1.93 = 148.07$ ml water needed

Final Answer: 50 ml D_{50}, 1.925 ml NaCl 4 mEq/ml and 148.07 ml water are needed.

❖ PRACTICE PROBLEMS

For the following problems, your pharmacy has on hand: 70% dextrose solution, sterile water, NaCl 4 mEq/ml and bupivacaine 0.5% solution.

Create the following solutions:

1. 200 ml (0.2 L) D_{10} ¼ NS
2. 1500 ml of ½ NS
3. 500 ml of D_{25} ¾ NS
4. 250 ml of D_{30}
5. 750 ml of D_{15} ⅓ NS
6. 100 ml of 0.0625% bupivacaine
7. 100 ml of 0.125% bupivacaine and 10 ml of fentanyl solution

146 *Percentage Preparations*

8. 1000 ml of D_6 ¼ NS
9. 900 ml of ¾ NS
10. 600 ml of D_{15} ½ NS

Create the following w/w calculations: (List how much of each ingredient is needed.)
11. 0.01% codeine in lactose—100 grams
12. 1% hydrocortisone in talc—50 grams
13. 5% zinc oxide in lanolin—20 grams
14. 0.5% hydrocortisone in talc—100 grams
15. 7% ferric oxide in lanolin—100 grams

For the following problems, you are given these stock preparations:

        Hydrocortisone cream 1%
        Dextrose in water 70%
        Sterile water
        Bupivacaine 0.5%
        Atropine in lactose 0.001 %
        Dextrose in water 10%

Create the following: (List amounts of all ingredients used.)
16. 100 grams of 0.25% hydrocortisone cream using an inert cream base
17. 150 ml of D_{30} using D_{10}, and D_{70}
18. 300 ml of D_{50} using D_{70} and water
19. 200 ml of bupivacaine 0.1%
20. 3000 ml of D_{25} using D_{10} and D_{70}

How many grams of active drug are contained in the following percent preparations:
21. 1 kilogram of 0.001% atropine in lactose
22. 500 ml of D_{30}
23. 150 grams of 0.5% hydrocortisone cream
24. 1 ml of 0.5% bupivacaine
25. 800 ml of D_{10}

List the quantities of each solution needed to create the following:
26. 3500 ml of $D_{12.5}$ $\frac{1}{4}$ NS using D_{70}, sterile water and NaCl 4 mEq/ml.

27. 750 ml of D_{40} $\frac{1}{2}$ NS using D_{70}, water and NaCl 4 mEq/ml.

28. 1 Liter of D_5 $\frac{1}{16}$ NS using D_{70}, water and NaCl 4 mEq/ml.

Chapter 20
PHARMACY ECONOMICS

In this chapter:
- *Why Pharmacy Economics?*
- *Calculating Percentage Markup*
- *Using Fees to Determine Price*

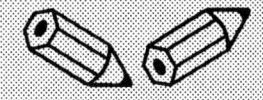

WHY PHARMACY ECONOMICS?

Although the pharmacy technicians deal primarily with the formation and delivery of medications, they must also pay some attention to the fiscal management policies which keep the pharmacy in business.

Often, the responsibility for purchasing and pricing medications is delegated to a technician. In order to be comfortable in such a position, the technician must be familiar with the information contained in this chapter.

Points to Remember

- The foundation of most pharmacy pricing strategies is AWP—"Average Wholesale Price."
- The AWP is actually an imaginary price created for the industry by the publishers of the Blue Book.
- The AWP is formulated from the manufacturer's selling price with an 18% markup.

CALCULATING PERCENTAGE MARKUPS
Understanding Acquisition Cost

The **acquisition cost** is the amount that the pharmacy actually has to pay the manufacturer for the medication. The acquisition cost is almost always less than AWP because of the effect of volume discounts, buying groups or wholesale contracts.

Buying groups are organizations formed for the primary purpose of extracting better prices from manufacturers. These groups are organized similarly to clubs in that pharmacies who wish to join the buying group pay for the privilege. The benefit of joining a buying group is that the buying group can negotiate much larger rebates and other discounts than any individual pharmacy ever could. The buying group has great negotiating power because its member pharmacists represent vast amounts of business to the manufacturer that presents the best prices.

Each type of pharmacy tends to belong to a buying group comprised mostly of pharmacies of that same type. For example, a hospital will most likely join a buying group that is composed mostly of hospitals, whereas a retail pharmacy will tend to join a buying group composed primarily of other retail pharmacies

Once a pharmacy has acquired a drug product, a price for the item must be determined. This price must be sufficient to cover all costs of running the pharmacy and, if the pharmacy is a for-profit organization, it must include a reasonable profit. There are several methods of determining selling price, but a discussion of any of them requires familiarity with some common terms.

Calculating Markup

The markup of an item is the amount (usually stated as a percentage) that is charged in addition to the cost of the medication. The following formula is used to calculate the price of a medication including the markup:

$$\text{Cost} \times 1.??$$

The above formula condenses several steps into one:

a. The 1 in 1. ?? gives a value equal to the cost of the medication

$$(\text{Cost} \times 1 = \text{cost})$$

b. The .?? in 1. ?? adds the markup (expressed as a decimal) to the cost

Some typical markups and how they fit into the formula are shown below:

Markup	Formula
200%	Cost × 3
300%	Cost × 4
10%	Cost × 1.1

The size of the markup is determined by the types of additional services provided with the medication, such as delivery, charge accounts, the volume of business and competition. The most common percentage markups in retail pharmacy are 33 ⅓ % and 50%, but others are used occasionally. Hospital pharmacy markups are typically much higher (200-400%) because of the inherent differences between retail and hospital pharmacies. Hospital pharmacies typically must generate large amounts of revenue to pay for services which the hospital provides but for which it does not bill. Examples of such services include security, housekeeping, utilities, nursing and respiratory care and administration. Hospitals must also keep a supply of many medications which are not frequently used, many of which expire and are disposed of without being used. Additionally, many hospitals give care to individuals who cannot or will not pay for treatment; therefore, other patients must pay for them.

✍ CHECK YOUR UNDERSTANDING

Calculate the final price of a 10 dollar item having a 33% markup:

a. Cost × 1.?? = price

b. 10 × 1.33 = 13.30

Answer: 13 dollars, 30 cents

Gross Margin

The difference between the final price and the acquisition cost is known as the **gross margin**. The gross margin must be sufficient to pay salaries, benefits, taxes, etc.

✍ CHECK YOUR UNDERSTANDING

What is the gross margin on an item which costs $10.00 and sells for $15.00?

a. Gross margin = Final price − acquisition cost

b. Gross margin = $15.00 − $10.00

Answer: $5.00

After all expenses have been deducted from the price, the remaining money is called the **net profit**. The expenses which must be deducted before net profit is determined include, but are not limited to, shipping fees, fixed costs such as rent and electricity, selling costs, wages, and the acquisition cost of the medication.

✍ CHECK YOUR UNDERSTANDING

An item sells for $15.00. If all expenses involved in the selling of the medication total $14.00, what is the net profit?

a. Net profit = Selling price − all expenses

b. Net profit = $15.00 − $14.00 − $1.00

Answer: $1.00

USING FEES TO DETERMINE PRICE
Pharmacy Fee

A pharmacy may use a **pharmacy fee** system rather than basing price on AWP plus a markup. The pharmacy fee system simply adds a set fee (often called a **dispensing fee**) to the cost of a medication. This fee may be the same regardless of the price of the medication, or it may vary according to the acquisition cost. The fee is designed to cover the cost of dispensing the item, including wages, delivery, rent, etc.

If the pharmacy fee varies according to price, the fee will normally increase as the acquisition cost increases:

Acquisition Cost	Pharmacy Fee
0-$9.99	$4.00
$10-$19.99	$6.00
$20-29.99	$7.00
$30 and above	$8.00

Another type of pricing system utilizes a percent markup plus a dispensing fee. The markup is supposed to cover the cost of the drug including inventory, storage, shipping, advertising, rent and other costs. The fee is intended to cover the labor cost of the pharmacist for his or her professional services.

Clinical Services Fee

A type of fee that did not exist until recently is the fee for clinical services. Instead of charging the patient for the delivery of a medication, this fee is generated from cognitive services provided by the pharmacist. This can range from instructing patients on how to use inhalers properly in the treatment of asthma to advising physicians on the most appropriate dose of a medication based on disease and organ function. Traditional fee systems are not appropriate for charging for delivery of clinical services because the product provided is not a manufactured item, but a result of the pharmacist's knowledge.

As this type of fee is relatively new, all ways of determining it have probably not yet been determined. Currently, some of the following ways of determining this fee are as follows:

- The fee is calculated based on savings to the patient. For example, if a pharmacist's intervention saves the patient $400.00, the clinical services fee would be $100.00.

- The fee is calculated based on the cost of providing the service, i.e. wages and benefits of the pharmacist providing the information.

Diagnosis Fee

Another type of fee system used primarily by the government is the diagnosis fee. All the known disease states and complications have been assigned a dollar amount that represents the average cost of treating a patient with that disease or complication plus a profit. The government will pay only that dollar amount regardless of how much it actually costs to treat the patient.

❖ PRACTICE PROBLEMS

1. What does the abbreviation AWP designate?
2. What is acquisition cost?
3. What is a buying group?
4. 100 capsules of tetracycline are acquired by a pharmacy for $10.00. If these tablets are then marked up 33 1/3% for sale, what is the final price?
5. Using the information in question 4, what would be the final price if a 50% markup were used?
6. What is the gross margin on those 100 capsules if they sell $15.00 and the acquisition cost is $10.00?
7. If the gross margin on a product is $10.00 and the final price is $30.00, what is the acquisition cost?
8. 30 procardia XL 30 mg tablets sell for $50.00. What is the net profit if the acquisition cost is $38.00 and all expenses add up to $11.00?
9. What is the difference between a pharmacy fee pricing system and a percentage markup?
10. Why are traditional pricing systems inappropriate methods of charging for the provision of clinical services?

ANSWER KEY

Chapter 9, The Language of Pharmacy

1. ss,I,V,X,L,C,D,M; **2**. **a.** 15; **b.** $4\frac{1}{2}$; **c.** 9; **d.** 35; **e.** 1,145; **f.** 145; **g.** 14; **h.** 490; **i.** $15\frac{1}{2}$;

3. **a.** n.p.o.; **b.** ac; **c.** pr; **d.** tsp; **e.** a.u.; **f.** q.i.d.; **g.** t.i.d.; **h.** q.d.; **i.** b.i.d.; **j.** gtt; **4. a.** XXIII; **b.** XVI; **c.** LV; **d.** IC; **e.** CVI; **f.** DI; **g.** DL; **h.** CM; **i.** MC; **j.** MM; **k.** MMM D; **6. a.** 21; **b.** 40; **c.** 66; **d.** 90; **e.** 166; **f.** 250; **g.** 1,010; **h.** 1,060; **i.** 540; **j.** 490; **k.** 2010

Chapter 10, Fractions

1. $\frac{1}{6}$; 2. $1\frac{1}{7}$; 3. $\frac{3}{10}$; 4. $\frac{3}{9}$; 5. $\frac{1}{13}$; 6. **a.** $\frac{3}{6}$ or $\frac{1}{2}$; **b.** $\frac{7}{16}$; **c.** $\frac{6}{21}$ or $\frac{2}{7}$; **d.** $\frac{21}{8}$ or $2\frac{5}{8}$; 7. $\frac{42}{49}$;

8. $\frac{1}{4}$; 9. **a.** $\frac{5}{16}$; **b.** $\frac{5}{56}$; **c.** $\frac{16}{9}$; **d.** $\frac{13}{16}$; 10. $\frac{7}{3}$; 11. $3\frac{1}{5}$; 12. $\frac{125}{1000}$ or $\frac{1}{8}$; 13. $\frac{45}{100}$ or $\frac{9}{20}$; 14. $3\frac{8}{17}$

15. $\frac{5}{6}$; **b.** $\frac{165}{112}$ or $1\frac{53}{112}$; 16. **a.** $\frac{121}{300}$; **b.** $\frac{29}{80}$; 17. **a.** $\frac{8}{27}$; **b.** $\frac{22}{105}$; 18. **a.** $\frac{18}{16}$ or $\frac{9}{8}$ or $1\frac{1}{8}$ **b.** $\frac{15}{5}$ or 3

Chapter 11, The Metric System

1. kilogram; 2. microliter 3. dekameter; 4. picogram; 5. pcg or pg; 6. ml; 7. km; 8. dl; 9. ng; 10. cm; 11. 1.5 km; 12. 40 l; 13. 8 kg; 14. 0.1 gram; 15. 0.125 mg

Chapter 12, Apothecaries' and Avoirdupois

1. 3.29 lb (avoir) or 3 lb, 4 ounces, 290 gr; **2.** 8.51 tb (apoth); **3.** gr 28437.5 or gr 26250; 4. 25 ml; **5.** 946 ml; **6.** 378.5 fl.oz. or 384 fl.oz. **7.** 26250 mg or 28437.5 mg; 8. 650 mg or 600 mg; **9.** 6 tsp or 5.914 tsp; **10.** 2 tsp; **11.** gr 2 or gr 2.17; **12.** 2 tbsp 13. 325 mg or 300 mg; **14.** 2 lb (avoir); **15.** 2.43 lb (apoth); **16.** 150 ml; **17.** 6500 mg or 6000 mg

Chapter 14, Ratio and Proportion
Ratio and Proportion

1. 66; 2. 182.95; 3. 31,680; 4. 126; 5. 2.5; **6.** 10 ml; **7.** 20 ml; **8.** 5; **9.** 6; **10. a.** 2.5 ml; **b.** 10 ml; **c.** 100 ml; **d.** 160 ml; **11.** 5 shelves (one shelf is partially filled); **12.** 30; 13. 4050 dollars; **14.** 5 ml; **15.** 13 tables (one table will have fewer than 10 guests); 16. 3 cases; **17.** 7875 yen; **18.** 62.5 ml; **19.** 6 tons; **20.** 9 grams; **21.** $333\frac{1}{3}$ g codeine, $666\frac{2}{3}$ g lactose; **22.** $333\frac{1}{3}$ g hydrocortisone, $166\frac{2}{3}$ g talc; **23.** $\frac{5}{6}$ mg folic acid, $4\frac{1}{6}$ sucrose; **24.** 25 grams dinoprostone, 75 grams surgilube; **25.** $1\frac{1}{2}$ pounds apples, $2\frac{1}{2}$ pounds oranges; **26.** $\frac{3}{2} = \frac{5}{9}$, 27 ≠ 10 (no equivalency);

154 Answers

27. $\frac{5}{10} = \frac{9}{18}$, 90 = 90 (Equivalency exists)

Methods of Calculation

  1. a. 1800; **b.** 6.5; **c.** 950; **2. a.** 3210; **b.** 100; **3.** 150

Chapter 14, Rounding

  1. 0.124; **2.** 0.26; **3.** 0.7; **4.** 1.61; **5.** 2.778; **6.** 1.252; **7.** 0.86; **8.** 0.12; **9.** 1.4; **10.** 127.189; **11.** 1.36; **12.** 50.1; **13.** 5.2468; **14.** 2.171; **15.** 3.92

Chapter 15, Dosing

  1. 2.5 ml; **2.** 5 ml; **3.** 7.5 ml; **4.** 2 ml; **5.** 4 ml; **6.** 15 ml; **7.** 10 ml; **8.** 10 ml; **9.** 20 ml; **10.** 20 ml; **11.** 2 ml; **12.** 2.5 ml; **13.** 5 ml; **14.** 10 ml; **15.** 3 ml; **16.** 1 ml; **17.** 0.25 ml; **18.** 2.5 ml; **19.** 70 mg; **20.** 70 mg; **21.** 106 mg; **22.** 140 mg; **23.** 180 mg; **24.** 136 mg; **25.** 190.9 mg; **26.** 202 mg; **27.** 5; **28.** 3; **29.** 40 tablets; **30.** 140 ml; **31.** 10.5 ml/hr; **32.** 18 ml/hr; **33.** 30 ml/hr; **34.** 150 ml; **35.** 25 drops/min; **36.** 31.25 drops/min; **37.** 100 ml/hour; **38.** 250 ml/hr; **39.** 3; **40.** 4; **41.** 5; **42.** 3; **43.** 5; **44.** 3; **45.** 3; **46.** $\frac{1}{2}$; **47.** 10 ml; **48.** 2.5 ml; **49.** 6 ml; **50.** 2.5 ml; **51.** 6 ml; **52.** 10 ml; **53.** 2.5 ml; **54.** 2.5 ml; **55.** 3 ml; **56.** 0.1 ml; **57.** 0.5 ml; **58.** 1.5 ml; **59.** 120 mg; **60.** 12.27 mg; **61.** 3600 mg; **62.** 2200 mg; **63.** 8.5 mg; **64.** appropriate; **65.** inappropriate; **66.** appropriate; **67.** appropriate; **68.** inappropriate; **69.** 1.5 mg; **70.** 80 mg

Chapter 16, Miscellaneous Calculations

Insulin Measurement

  1. 0.1 ml; **2.** 0.2 ml; **3.** 0.3 ml; **4.** 0.6 ml; **5.** 0.8 ml; **6.** 0.9 ml; **7.** 2 ml; **8.** 1.5 ml; **9.** 1 ml; **10.** 0.9 ml; **11.** 0.9 ml; **12.** 0.4 ml; **13.** 0.5 ml; **14.** 0.3 ml; **15.** 0.2 ml

Temperature Conversions

  1. -17.8° C; **2.** -12.2° C; **3.** 6.7° C; **4.** 0° C; **5.** 10° C; **6.** 22.2° C; **7.** 32.2° C; **8.** 43.3° C; **9.** 65.6° C; **10.** 73.9° C; **11.** 100° C; **12.** 148.9° C; **13.** -41.8° F; **14.** -4° F; **15.** 23° F; **16.** 32° F; **17.** 50° F; **18.** 77° F; **19.** 100.4° F; **20.** 105.8° F; **21.** 113° F; **22.** 221° F

Automatic Compounders

  1. 0.88; **2.** 2; **3.** 292.5 g; **4.** 450 g; **5.** 1.1; **6.** 825.5 mg; **7.** No, the weight should be 234 grams; **8.** 1120 grams; **9.** 1116 grams; **10.** 757.5 grams; **11.** 220 grams; **12.** 1.2; **13.** 2; **14.** 1; **15.** 1.1; **16.** 4

Chapter 17, Dilutions

  1. 0.5 ml ondansetron stock dilute to 100 ml (Each dose = 0.1 ml); **2.** 5 ml gentamicin stock dilute to 20 ml; **3.** 0.5 ml of Digoxin stock dilute to 5 ml; **4.** 1 ml of metoclopramide stock; **5.** 0.4 ml morphine stock, dilute to 4 ml; **6.** 2 ml nafcillin stock; **7.** 2.5 ml dexamethasone stock; **8.** 0.1 ml of gentamicin stock, dilute to 2 ml; **9.** 1 ml nafcillin stock, dilute to 10 ml; **10. a.** 0.5 ml stock, dilute to 2 ml; **b.** same as a (0.2 ml will be wasted); **c.** 0.4 ml stock, dilute to 1.6 ml; **d.** 0.3 ml stock, dilute to 1.2 ml; **11. a.** 0.1 ml stock, dilute to 500 ml; **b.** 0.1 ml

stock, dilute to 200 ml; **c.** 0.1 ml stock, dilute to 100 ml; **d.** 0.3 ml stock, dilute to 100 ml; **e.** 0.1 ml stock, dilute to 5 ml; **f.** 0.1 ml stock; **g.** 0.3 ml stock; **h.** 0.5 ml (no dilution)—Obviously, with this type of dilution, there is a great amount of unavoidable wastage;
12. 0.6 ml stock

Chapter 18, Electrolyte Calculations

1. 3 ml; **2.** 20 meq; **3.** 320 mg; **4.** 55.85 mg; **5.** 4.8 ml NaCl and 245.2 ml water; **6.** 57.8 ml NaCl and 1,142.2 ml water; **7.** 14.4 ml NaCl and 735.6 ml water; **8.** 6.4 ml NaCl and 493.6 ml water; **9.** 5.8 ml NaCl and 294.2 ml water; **10.** 3.9 ml NaCl and 396.1 ml; **11.** 36.5 mg; **12.** 30 meq, **13.** 832.7 mg; **14.** 1,193 mg; **15.** 20 ml

Chapter 19, Percentage Preparations

1. 28.57 or 28.6 ml D_{70}, 1.92 ml NaCl 4 mEq/ml and 169.51 ml sterile water; **2.** 28.87 ml of NaCl 4 mEq/ml, 1471.13 ml sterile water; **3.** 178.57 ml D_{70}, 14.43 ml NaCl 4 mEq/ml, 307 ml sterile water; **4.** 107.14 ml D_{70}, 142.85 ml sterile water; **5.** 160.71 ml D_{70}, 9.62 ml NaCl 4 mEq/ml, 579.67 ml sterile water; **6.** 12.5 ml bupivacaine 0.5%, 87.5 ml diluent;
7. 25 ml bupivacaine 0.5%, 65 ml diluent **8.** 85.71 ml D_{70}, 9.63 ml NaCl 4 mEq/ml, 904.66 ml sterile water; **9.** 25.99 ml NaCl 4 mEq/ml, 874.01 ml sterile water; **10.** 128.57 ml D_{70}, 11.55 ml NaCl, 4mEq/ml, 459.88 ml sterile water; **11.** 0.01 grams or 10 milligrams codeine and 99.99 grams lactose; **12.** 0.5 grams or 500 milligrams hydrocortisone, and 49.5
13. 1 gram zinc oxide, 19 grams lanolin; **14.** 0.5 grams hydrocortisone, 99.5 grams talc,
15. 7 grams ferric oxide, 93 grams lanolin; **16.** 50 grams 1% hydrocortisone cream, 50 grams cream base; **17.** 50 ml D_{70}, 100ml D_{10}, **18.** 214.29 ml D_{70}, 85.71 ml water;
19. 40 ml bupivacaine, 160 ml water; **20.** 750 ml D_{70}, 2,250 ml D_{10}; **21.** 0.01 grams (or 10 mg) atropine; **22.** 150 grams dextrose; **23.** 0.75 grams (or 750 mg) hydrocortisone; **24.** 5 mg bupivacaine; **25.** 80 grams dextrose; **26.** 625 ml D_{70}, 33.69 ml NaCl 4 meq/ml, 2841.3 ml water; **27.** 428.59 ml D_{70}, 14.44 ml NaCl 4 meq/ml, 306.99 ml water; **28.** 71.43 ml D_{70}, 2.4 ml NaCl 4 meq/ml, 926.17 ml water

Chapter 20, Pharmacy Economics

1. Average wholesale price; **2.** Acquisition cost is the actual price a pharmacy must pay to acquire a medication; **3.** A buying group is an organization whose purpose is to obtain a favorable pricing from drug manufacturers; **4.** $13.33 (1.333 × $10.00);
5. $15.00 (1.5 × $10.00); **6.** $5.00 ($15.00 − $10.00); **7.** $20.00
{Final price − acquisition = gross margin; $30.00 − ? = 10.00;
$30.00 − $10.00 = $20.00}; **8.** $1.00; **9.** The pharmacy fee is a set fee; it does not vary automatically according to acquisition cost; **10.** Because there is no tangible product, traditional fee schedules do not have a base from which to work

INDEX

♣ A

Abbreviations, 75
Absorption, 2-3
Acetaminophen, 22
Acetic acid, 31
Acetohexamide, 42
Acetylcholine, 29-30
Aqueous humor, 34
Acquisition cost, 148, 150
Activated partial thromboplastin time (aPTT), 14
Acyclovir, 11, 32
Addison's disease, 38
Adrenal hormones, 38
Agranulocytosis, 26
Air, 7
Alfentanyl HCl, 22
Aliquot, 125
Alligation, 142
Alprazolam, 27
Aluminum, 131
Aluminum carbonate, 34
Aluminum hydroxide, 34
Aluminum magnesium combinations, 34
Aluminum phosphate, 34
Aluminum sulfate, 33
Amantadine, 12
Aminophylline, 45, 113
Amiodarone HCl, 15
Amitriptyline, 25
Amlodipine besylate, 18
Amobarbital, 28
Amoxapine, 25
Amoxicillin trihydrate, 10
Ampicillin, 10
Amphotericin B, 6, 11
Ampule, 64-66, 68
Analgesic effects, 20
Androgens, 39
Angina, 19
Angiotensin II, 17
Angiotensin-converting enzyme (ACE) inhibitor, 17
Antacids, 34
Anti-infective agents, 11
Anti-infective drugs, 10
Anti-inflammatory agents, 21, 38
Antiarrhythmics, 15
Anticoagulants, 13
Anticonvulsants, 23
Antidepressant agents, 24
Antiemetics, 37
Antihistamines, 9, 37
Antihypertensive drugs, 16
Antimicrobial agents, 10
Antineoplastic drugs, 12
Antipsychotic, 37
Antipyretic effects, 20
Apothecaries' system, 89
Apraclonidine, 29
Argon, 131, 134
Ascorbic acid, 47
Aseptic technique, 53-54, 59-60
Aspirin, 20
Astemizole, 9
Atenolol, 16
Antineoplastic medications, 55, 67
Atomic weight, 130-132
Atracurium besylate, 46
Atria, 14
Augmented betamethasone, 33
Automatic compounders, 122
Average wholesale price, 147
Avoirdupois system, 89
Aztreonam, 10

♣ B

b.i.d., 74
Bacitracin, 29
Baclofen, 46
Bacteria, 10
Bacterial contamination, 53, 59
Barbiturates, 27-28
Benazepril, 17
Benzocaine, 31, 33, 43
Benzocaine/antipyrine, 31
Benzocaine/phenol, 31
Benzodiazepines, 27-28
Benzoyl peroxide, 31
Bepridil HCl, 18
Beta carotene, 47
Betamethasone, 33, 38
Betaxolol, 29
Bile, 3
Biological safety cabinets (BSCs), 55, 58, 67
Biotransformation, 2
Bisacodyl, 36
Bleomycin, sulfate, 12
Body surface area (BSA), 105
Brain, 20
Brevicon, 41
Brompheniramine, 10
BSC pump
    Type A, 55
    Type B, 55
Bumetanide, 16
Bupivacaine HCl, 43

Bupropion, 25
Busulfan, 12
Butorphanol tartrate, 22

♣ C

Calcifediol, 47
Calciferol, 48
Calcitriol, 47
Calcium, 131
Calcium carbonate, 34
Calcium-channel blocking agents, 18
Captopril, 17
Carbachol, 29-30
Carbamazepine, 23
Carbamide peroxide, 31
Carbon, 131
Carboplatin, 12
Cardiovascular drugs, 14
Carisoprodol, 46
Carteolol, 29
Cascara sagrada, 36
Castor oil, 36
Cefazolin sodium, 10
Cefotaxime sodium, 10
Cefoxitin sodium, 10
Ceftriaxone sodium, 10
Cefuroxime sodium, 10
Cellufresh, 31
Celluvise, 31
Central nervous system, 20
Centrally-acting agents, 19
Cephalexin, 10
Cetylpyridinium, 31
Chemotherapeutic agents (see also Antineoplastic agents), 12-13
Chemotherapy, 67
Chlorambucil, 12
Chloramphenicol, 29, 31
Chlordiazepoxide, 27
Chlorhexidine gluconate, 31
Chlorine, 131
Chloroprocaine, 43
Chlorpheniramine, 9-10
Chlorpromazine, 26
Chlorpropamide, 42
Chlorzoxazone, 46
Ciclopirox olamine, 32
Cimetidine, 37
Ciprofloxacin, 29
Cisplatin, 12
Class 100, 54
Clindamycin, 31
Clinical services fee, 150
Clobetasol propionate, 33
Clomipramine, 25
Clonazepam, 23
Clonidine HCl, 19
Clotrimazole, 11, 31
Clozapine, 26

Co-trimoxazole, 10
Coal tar, 32
Cocaine, 43, 46
Codeine, 22
Colloid, 6
Compatibilities, 6, 67
Compatibility information, 7
Compounder, 123
Consistency
    Change of consistency, 7
Constant infusions, 112
Constipation, 36
Container
    Hermetic, 8
    Immediate, 8
    Light-resistant, 8
    Tamper-resistant, 8
    Tight, 8
    Well-closed, 8
Contamination, 60
Conversions, 132
Copper, 131
Creams, 5
Curare, 47
Cyanocobalamin, 47
Cyclopentolate, 30
Cyclophosphamide, 12
Cytarabine, 12

♣ D

Dacarbazine, 12
Danazol, 39
Dantrolene sodium, 46
Daunorubicin, 12
Decomposition, 67
Decongestants, 10
Demulen, 41
Desipramine, 25
Dexamethasone, 29, 38
Dexbrompheniramine, 10
Dextroamphetamine, 28
Dextromethorphan hydrobromide, 31
Diabetes, 41
Diagnosis fee, 150
Diazepam, 23, 27
Dibucaine, 33
Diclofenac, 20, 30
Didanosine, 11
Dienestrol, 40
Diethylstilbestrol, 40
Diflunisal, 20
Digoxin, 15
Dihydrotachysterol, 47
Dihydroxyaluminum sodium carbonate, 34
Diltiazem HCl, 18
Dilutions, 125
Dimenhydrinate, 9, 37
Dimensional analysis, 87
Diphenhydramine, 9

Diphenhydramine/calamine, 32
Diphenoxylate with atropine, 35
Dipivefrin, 29-30
Disopyramide, 15
Dispensing fee, 149
Distribution, 2-3
Diuretics, 16
Divalproex, 23
Docusate calcium, 36
Docusate sodium, 36
Dosage forms, 5
Dosage range, 104
Dosing, 104
    Capsules, 108
    Constant infusions, 113
    Liquids, 108
    Tablets, 108
Dosing chart
    Adult body surface area chart, 105
    Children's body surface area chart, 105
Doxazosin maleate, 19
Doxepin, 25
Doxorubicin, 12
Doxycycline, 10
Droperidol, 13
Drug additive transfer, 65
Drug forms
    Capsules, 5
    Chewable tablets, 5
    Elixirs, 5
    Solutions, 5
    Suspensions, 5
    Tablets, 5
Drug storage of, 8
Drugs,
    Metabolites of, 3
Ductus arteriosus, 21
Dyphylline, 45

♣ E

Echothiophate, 30
Electrolytes, 129
Elements, 131
Elimination, 4
Emollients, 33
Enalapril maleate, 17
Encainide, 15
Enoxaparin, 14
Epinephrine, 29-30
Equivalent weight, 130
Ergocalciferol, 47
Erythromycin, 10, 29, 31
Esmolol, 16
Estradiol, 40
Estrogenic substances, conjugated, 40
Estrogens, 39-40
Etidocaine, 43
Etodolac, 20
Excretion, 3

Excretion, 2
Expiration date, 7
Extrapyramidal symptoms (EPS), 27

♣ F

Famotidine, 37
Feces, 3
Felbamate, 23
Felodipine, 18
Fentanyl citrate, 22
Filgrastim, 13
Flavoxate HCl, 44
Flecainide acetate, 15
Flexible plastic containers, 51
Flexible plastic intravenous container, 65
Fluorine, 131
5-Fluorouracil, 12
Fluconazole, 11
Fludarabine phosphate, 12
Fludrocortisone acetate, 38
Flunisolide, 38
Fluocinolone, 33
Fluocinonide, 33
Fluoxetine, 25
Fluoxymesterone, 39
Fluphenazine, 26
Flurazepam, 27
Flurbiprofen, 30
Folate, 47
Follicle-stimulating hormone-releasing factor, 41
Fosinopril, 17
Fractions, 96
Freezing, protection from, 8
Fungi, 10
Furosemide, 16

♣ G

Gabapentin, 23
Gastrointestinal agents, 37
Gastrointestinal system, 34
Gentamicin sulfate, 10, 29, 32
Glaucoma, 34
Glipizide, 42
Glucocorticoid effects, 38
Glyburide, 42
Gold, 131
Grams, 132
Granisetron, 13
Griseofulvin, 11
Gross margin, 149
Guanabenz acetate, 19

♣ H

H2 Antagonists, 37
Half-life, 4
Haloperidol, 26
Helium, 131, 134

Hematoma, 14
Heparin, 14
High efficiency particulate air (HEPA) filter, 55, 58, 64-65
Histamine, 9
Homatropine, 30
Horizontal flow, 54
Hormones, 38
Household system, 91
Humidity, 7
Humulin, 41
Hydralazine HCl, 18
Hydrochlorothiazide, 16
Hydrocortisone, 33, 38
Hydrocortisone/acetic acid, 31
Hydrogen, 131
Hydromorphone HCl, 22
Hydroxyzine, 9
Hypertension, 16-19
Hypocalcemia, 48
Hypoglycemia, 42
Hypophosphatemia, 48
Hypotears, 31
Hypothalamus, 20, 41

✤ I

I.V. (continuous) infusion, 51, 52
I.V. push, 51
Ibuprofen, 20
Idarubicin, 12
Ifosfamide, 12
Iletin, 41
Imipramine, 25
Immune system, 3
Imipenem, 11
Incompatibilities, 6
Increased intraocular pressure (IOP), 34
Indomethacin, 20
Infection
    Barrier to, 3
Injections
    Epidural, 5
    Intra-arterial, 2, 51
    Intradermal, 3, 5, 51
    Intramuscular, 2, 5, 51
    Intrathecal, 5, 51
    Intravenous, 2, 5, 51
    Subcutaneous, 5, 51
    Insomnia, 27
Insulin, 38, 41
    Lente, 42, 120
    Measurement of, 120
    Mixed NPH/regular, 120
    NPH, 42, 120
    PZI, 120
    Regular, 42, 120
    Semilente, 120
    Ultralente, 42, 120
Intermittent (piggyback) infusion, 52

International Normalized Ratio (INR), 14
Intravenous infusions, 66
Iodine, 131
Iron, 131
Irrigation, 52
Irrigation bottles, 66
Isocarboxazid, 24
Isoflurophate, 30
Isopropyl alcohol/glycerin, 31
Isosorbide dinitrate, 18
Isosorbide mononitrate, 18
Isradipine, 18

✤ K

Kaolin and pectin, 35
Keratolytic, 33
Ketoconazole, 11
Ketoprofen, 20
Ketorolac, 20, 30
Kidneys, 3
Krypton, 134

✤ L

Label specifications, 7
Labeling, 66
Laminar airflow hoods, 54, 55, 60
Lanolin, 33
Laxatives, 36
Lead, 131
Leur-lock fittings, 68
Leur-lock tip, 61
Levobunolol, 29
Levothyroxine, 43
Lidocaine HCl, 15, 33, 43
Light, 7
Lindane, 32
Liothyronine, 43
Liotrix, 43
Lipophilic, 3
Liquifilm Forte, 31
Lisinopril, 17
Lithium, 26, 131
Local anesthetics, 13, 30, 43
Loperamide HCl, 35
Lorazepam, 27
Lotions, 5
Loxapine, 26

✤ M

Magaldrate, 35
Magnesium, 131
Magnesium citrate, 36
Magnesium hydroxide, 35-36
Magnesium salicylate/choline salicylate, 21
Malignant hyperthermia, 46
Maprotiline, 25

Meclizine, 9, 37
Medications, 5
    Acne, 31
    Burns, 31
    Ear, 31
    Mouth and throat, 31
    Topical, 31
Medroxyprogesterone, 40
Megestrol acetate, 40
Menadione, 48
Menthol, 31
Meperidine, 22
Mepivacaine HCl, 44
Mercury, 131
Mesoridazine, 26
Metabolism, 2-3
Methocarbamol, 46
Methotrexate, 12
Methychlothiazide, 16
Methylcellulose, 36
Methyldopa, 19
Methylphenidate, 28
Methylprednisolone, 38
Metipranolol, 29
Metoclopramide HCl, 13
Metoprolol tartrate, 16
Metric volume, 86
Metric abbreviations, 86
Metric length, 86
Metric measurement, 85
Metric terms, 85
Metric weight, 86
Metronidazole, 11
Mexiletine HCl, 15
Miconazole, 11, 32
Midazolam, 27
Milliequivalent, 130
Milligrams, 132
Mineral oil, 36
Mineralocorticoid effects, 38
Minoxidil, 19
Miotics, 29-30
Mitoxantrone, 13
Mitomycin, 12
Mixtard, 41
Monoamine-oxidase inhibitors (MAOIs), 24, 25
Morphine, 22
Mupirocin, 32
Muscle relaxants, 44
    Skeletal, 46
    Smooth, 44
    Smooth, respiratory, 45
Mydriatics, 29
Myocardial infarction, 19

♣ N

Nadolol, 16
Nafcillin, 11
Nalbuphine HCl, 22
Naphazoline, 30
Naproxen, 21
Needles, 60-61, 64-66
Needle shaft, 62
Neomycin/polymyxin, 11, 29
Neomycin/polymyxin B hydrocortisone, 31
Neon, 131, 134
Neuromuscular-blocking agents, 46
Neurotransmitters, 24
Niacin, 47
Nicardipine HCl,, 18
Nifedipine, 18
Nitrate-free period, 19
Nitrates, 19
Nitrofurazone, 32
Nitrogen, 131
Nitroglycerin, 19, 113
Nizatidine, 37
Nonpyrogenic, 3
Nonsteroidal anti-inflammatory agents (NSAIDs), 20, 21, 30
Norepinephrine, 24-25
Norethindrone, 40
Normal saline, 134
Nortriptyline, 25
Novolin, 41
Nystatin, 11, 31-32

♣ O

Ointments, 5
Omeprazole, 37
Ondansetron, 37
Ondansetron HCl, 13
Opiates, 21
Opium, 35
Oral contraceptives, 41
Oral drugs, 5
Orphenadrine citrate, 46
Ortho-Cept, 41
Ortho-Novum, 41
Ovral, 41
Oxaprozin, 21
Oxazepam, 27
Oxybutynin, 44
Oxycodone HCl, 22
Oxygen, 131
Oxymetazoline, 30
Oxytriphylline, 45

♣ P

PO, 74
Paclitaxel, 13
Pain, 20
Pancuronium bromide, 46
Pantothenic acid, 47
Papaverine HCl, 19
Parenteral dosage forms, 5

Paroxetine, 25
Penicillin, 11
Pentazocine HCl, 22
Pentobarbital, 28
Percent strength, 138
Permethrin, 32
Perphenazine, 26
Personal attire, 60
Personnel, 59
Pharmacokinetics, 2-3
Pharmacy fee, 149-150
Phenelzine, 24
Phenobarbital, 23, 28
Phenol/menthol, 31
Phenolphthalein, 36
Phenylephrine, 30
Phenylpropanolamine, 10
Phenytoin, 23
Phosphorus, 131
Physostigmine, 29-30
Phytonadione, 48
Pilocarpine atropine, 29-30
Piperacillin sodium, 11
Piroxicam, 21
Platelets, 21
Podophyllum resin, 33
Polymyxin B/bacitracin, 32
Polymyxin B/neomycin/bacitracin, 32
Potassium, 16, 131
Potassium/sodium bicarbonate, 35
Potency, 7
Pound fraction, 92
Prazosin HCl, 19
Precipitates, 6
Precipitation, 67
Prednisolone, 29, 38
Prednisone, 38
Primidone, 23
Procainamide HCl, 15
Procaine, 44
Prochlorperazine, 13, 26, 37
Progestins, 39-40
Promethazine, 9, 13, 37
Proparacaine, 30
Proportion, 87, 97, 99
Proportion method, 96
Propoxyphene HCl, 22
Propranolol, 17
Prostaglandins, 20
Protective cap, 63
Prothrombin time (PT), 14
Protriptyline, 25
Pseudoephedrine, 10
Psychotropic agents, 26
Psyllium, 36
Pyridoxine, 47
Pyrogens, 3

♣ Q

Quinestrol, 40
Quinidine, 15
Quinine, 16

♣ R

Ramipril, 17
Ranitidine, 37
Rapid eye movement (R.E.M.) sleep, 27
Ratio, 99
Rectum, 3
Refrigeration, 7
Resperidone, 26
Ribavirin, 11
Riboflavin, 47
Rickets, 48
Rimantadine, 12
Roman numerals, 73
Routes of administration, 5, 6, 50
    Epidural, 6
    Intradermal, 6
    Intramuscular, 6
    Intravenous, 6
    Oral, 6
    Rectal, 6
    Subcutaneous, 6
    Sublingual, 6
    Topical, 6
    Transdermal, 6

♣ S

Salicylic acid, 33
Saline preparations, 134
Salsalate, 21
Schizophrenia, 26
Scopolamine, 30
Secobarbital, 28
Selenium sulfide, 32
Senna, 36
Serotonin, 24-25
Serotonin-uptake inhibitors, 24-25
Sertraline, 25
Sex hormones, 38-39
Silicon, 131
Silver, 131
Silver sulfadiazine, 32
Simethicone, 35
Sodium, 131
Sodium bicarbonate, 35
Sodium chloride, 134
Specific concentration dosing, 139
Specific gravity, 123
Spinal cord, 20
Spironolactone, 16
Stability, 7, 67
Sterile, 3

Sterile compounding area, 54
Sterile products, 50, 59, 67
Steroidal anti-inflammatory drugs, 33
Storage, 7
Storage areas, 7
Storage definitions, 8
Sublingual, 3, 5
Succinylcholine, 46
Sulfonylureas, 42
Sulindac, 21
Synapse, 24
Syringes, 61, 64-65, 66
Syringe caps, 66

✤ T

Tamoxifen, 13
Tannic acid, 31
Temazepam, 27
Temperature, 8
    Cold, 8
    Cool, 8
    Excessive heat, 8
    Freezer, 8
    Room temperature, 8
    Warm, 8
Terfenadine, 9
Testosterone, 39
Tetracaine, 30, 33, 44

Tetracycline HCl, 11, 29, 31
Tetrahydrozoline HCl, 30
Theophylline, 45
Therapeutic effect, 3
Thiamine, 47
Thioridazine, 26
Thiothixene, 26
Thyroglobulin, 43
Thyroid hormone, 43
    Natural, 43
    Synthetic, 43
Thyroid hormones, 38
Ticarcillin disodium, 11
Timolol maleate, 17, 29
Tobramycin sulfate, 11, 29
Tobramycin
Tolazamide, 42
Tolbutamide, 42
Tolmetin sodium, 21
Tolnaftate, 11, 32
Topical drugs, 29, 51
Tranylcypromine, 24
Trazodone, 25
Tretinoin, 31
Triamcinolone, 33, 38
Triamterene, 16
Triazolam, 27
Tricyclic antidepressants, 25

Tricyclic compounds, 24
Trifluoperazine, 26
Trimethobenzamide HCl, 13, 37
Trimipramine, 25
Triphasil, 41
Triprolidine, 10
Trolamine salicylate, 33
Tropicamide, 30

✤ U

Urine, 3

✤ V

Vagina, 3
Valence, 131-132, 134
Valproic acid, 23
Vancomycin HCl, 11
Vasodilating agents, 18
Vecuronium bromide, 46, 112
Ventricles, 14
Verapamil HCl, 18
Vertical flow, 54
Vial, 63-66, 68
Vidarubine, 11
Vinblastine sulfate, 13
Vincristine sulfate, 13
Viruses, 10
Vitamin A, 33
Vitamin D, 33
Vitamins, 47
    Fat-soluble, 47
    Water soluble, 47
Volume, 123

✤ W

Warfarin, 14

Wernicke-Korsakoff syndrome, 48

✤ X

Xenon, 134

✤ Z

Zalcitabine, 11
Zidovudine, 11
Zinc oxide, 33

Career Colleges/Community Colleges and Post Secondary Vo-Techs
For desk or review copies call: 1-800-477-3692 or fax 1-518-464-0301
For orders call: 1-800-347-7707 or fax 1-606-647-5023
Mail to: ITP Career Education
       Attn: Order Fulfillment
       P.O. Box 6904
       Florence, KY 41022
       Email: info@delmar.com

Four-Year College/University
For desk or review copies call: 1-800-423-0563 or fax 1-606-647-5020
For orders call: 1-800-354-9706 or fax 1-800-487-8488
Mail to: ITP Higher Education
       Attn: Order Fulfillment
       P.O. Box 6904
       Florence, KY 41022

Business, Industry and Government
For orders call: 1-800-347-7707, ext. 4 or fax 1-606-647-5963
Mail to: ITP Business, Industry, Government
       Attn: Order Fulfillment
       P.O. Box 6904
       Florence, KY 41022
       All other orders and inquiries
       1-800-347-7707, ext. 4

Retail
Mail to: International Thomson Publishing
       Attn: Professional/Technical Order Fulfillment
       P.O. Box 6904
       Florence, KY 41022
       Phone: 1-800-842-3636 or fax 1-606-647-5963

High Schools and Secondary Vo-techs
For desk or review copies call: 1-800-824-5179 or fax 1-800-453-7882
For orders call: 1-800-354-9706 or fax 1-800-487-8488
Mail to: ITP School
       Attn: Order Fulfillment
       P.O. Box 6904
       Florence, KY 41022

Canada
Mail to: Nelson ITP Canada
       1120 Birchmount Road
       Scarborough, Ontario M1K 5G4
       Canada
Telephone Number: 1-416-752-9448 or 1-800-268-2222
Fax Number: 1-416-752-8101 or 1-800-430-4445
E-mail: inquire@nelson.com

International Ordering
Mail to: International Thomson Learning
       P.O. Box 6904
       Florence, KY 41022
       Phone: 1-606-282-5786
       Fax: 1-606-282-5700